Bedlam

BEDLAM

A Year in the Life of a Mental Hospital

by Dominick Bosco

A Birch Lane Press Book
Published by Carol Publishing Company

A Birch Lane Press Book
Published by Carol Publishing Group
Birch Lane Press is a registered trademark of Carol Communications, Inc.
Editorial Offices: 600 Madison Avenue, New York, N.Y. 10022
Sales & Distribution Office: 120 Enterprise Avenue, Secaucus, N.J. 07094
In Canada: Canadian Manda Group, P.O. Box 920, Station U, Toronto
Ontario M8Z 5P9

Queries regarding rights and permissions should be addressed to Carol Publishing Group, 600 Madison Avenue, New York, N.Y. 10022

Carol Publishing Group books are available at special discounts for bulk purchases, for sales promotions, fund raising, or educational purposes. Special editions can be created to specifications. For details, contact: Special Sales Department, Carol Publishing Group, 120 Enterprise Avenue, Secaucus, N.J. 07094

Manufactured in the United States of America
10   9   8   7   6   5   4   3   2   1

Library of Congress Cataloging-in-Publication Data

Bosco, Dominick.
    Bedlam / by Dominick Bosco.
       p.   cm.
    "A Birch Lane Press book."
    ISBN 1–55972–113–8 (cloth) :
    1. Psychiatric hospitals—United States.   2. Psychiatric hospital patients—United States.   3. Mentally ill—Institutional care—United States—Case studies.   I. Title.
    [DNLM: 1. Hospitals, Psychiatric—popular works.   2. Mental Disorders—personal narratives.   3. Mental Disorders—popular works. WM 75 B742b]
    RC443.B67   1992
    362.2'1—dc20
    DNLM/DLC   91-47860
    for Library of Congress   CIP

For
All the mothers and fathers
And all the sons and daughters

And for
My Long Lost Secret Agent Brother:
If I gave back what I stole,
This would be a much smaller book.
But if I lost what you have given me,
My life would be much diminished.

There is a crime here that goes beyond denunciation. There is a sorrow here that weeping cannot symbolize. There is a failure here that topples all our success.

John Steinbeck
The Grapes of Wrath

This book, which is a work of nonfiction, attempts to represent the reality of life in a mental hospital for the patients, their families, and for the physicians and other professionals who care for the mentally ill.

Over the course of more than two years I conducted scores of interviews, mostly with members of one hospital community. I also talked with people from other institutions, as well as with friends and family members who are involved in the treatment or the experience of mental illness. What I quickly discovered was that there were recurring themes and details in many of their stories.

I was asked never to name the actual people interviewed or the institutions investigated, since the fear of reprisal is very great. I have respected the privacy of my sources, for two reasons—first, because I became convinced that their fears were justified, second, because my goal was not to expose any particular institution.

All of the events and conversations in this book were recounted to me by persons who did witness or participate in them. The thoughts of now deceased patients were constructed from discussions with their physicians and other caregivers and from medical records that included interviews with and statements by the patients. The entire text has been reviewed for accuracy by the actual sources.

I do not offer this book as a "balanced" piece of journalism. I am, to the best of my abilities, faithfully reporting what I saw and heard.

Dominick Bosco

ACKNOWLEDGMENTS

My deepest appreciation to the many people who helped with this book. To those who sat many hours with me and told me their stories: I wish I could give your real names. Instead, thank you Fran Channing and Alex Greco for the many doors you opened.

Thank you Woodrow Benjamin Rush, Wendy Dixon Billings, George Konopski, Steven and Ethel Rose, Faith Dundee, and Dolores Woods for guiding me once those doors were opened.

Thank you, Lily Speere, for sharing that bus ride with me.

I am also indebted to the many members of the National Alliance for the Mentally Ill who took precious time away from the good work they are doing and told me their stories. Also, many members and staff of the American Psychiatric Association provided invaluable assistance.

I am also grateful to:

Russell Galen, whose imagination helped inspire this book, and whose loyalty helped sustain it;

Nick Bakalar and Harvey Plotnick, for the low-interest loan that helped support the writing of the book until a publisher could be found;

Steve Schragis for being that publisher;

Gail Kinn, my editor, for her enthusiasm and caring guidance, and for all those encouraging words that are so important.

I am also indebted to Eileen Ebner and all the people at Wordstar, for a wonderful tool second to none.

And to my friends and family, who have listened to my ramblings from the very first, fed me, comforted me, and made sure I always had a home: Charles Gerras, Jack and Marianne Goodwin, Jim Gibson and Deborah Rouse, Michael Lafavore and Trieste Kennedy and Nico, John Feltman and Jean Rogers, Leslie and Barbara Lang and Jonathan, Mary Ann and Mark Lassen and Malery and Seth, Dr. Robert Berley and Gail and Alissa and Matthew, Sandy and Harry Lederman, Diane Raymond, Susan Zilber, Kathy and Shannon Eagan, Peg O'Shea, Kris Bennett, Patti Reed, Bill Hartwell, Mary Sue Welsh, Sara Forster, Gus Weinke, Linda Tyree, and, of course, Emma and Joe, Lore and Steve and Teri, Marianne, Sunny, and Bonne, and the Boscos of Trapani, especially Salvatore.

Bedlam

1 _____

[1]

For a few moments before she was fully awake, the first light of
morning was a pure light for Fran Channing. The sky was clean, and
the day was a sweet blessing that made her heart swell with promise
as it had when she was a child on summer mornings. But she was
not fully conscious yet, and as she blinked and stirred she also
remembered, and her heart withered. She was not a little girl, and it
was not summer. The bright winter sun, baking sheets and blankets
through the window glass, had a way of fooling her. As a child she
would touch her fingers to the pane to make sure. Now she had no
need to do that, she could see the ice. Sun or no, a quarter-inch-
thick layer of ice had grown up the bottoms of the windows during
the night.

Fran lay still, tried not to see the ice, and stared into the sky.

She remembered a morning just like this one, a few days after
New Year's, a decade ago, the last morning of her life she would
ever allow herself that girlish sense of joy at the uncluttered good-

1

ness of a new day. That morning, Fran had awakened with it, as she often did, but then had come the smudge, the handprint of disaster blurred across the blue sky.

At first Fran thought it was just a general foreboding because her son Walter was to go back to college that day.

What a pathetic sight he had been a month earlier on the open train platform the night he arrived from school, lugging his steamer trunk, Brad's tattered old suitcase from the war, his guitar case, and a canvas bag stuffed with three weeks' worth of laundry. It was snowing all over the boy, covering his shoulders and head. The flakes blended in with his bushy hair and eyebrows and gave him the look of an old man.

This memory particularly stung Fran because although he was now only twenty-seven, Walter had real gray hair and a map of wrinkles across the pallor of his face.

Walter had started to cry when he saw them coming and had thrown his arms around each of them, murmuring their names under breath heavy with sobs. The three of them embraced on the train platform, one week before Christmas, nine years and a few weeks ago. The wind blew the cold between them and under their coats as Brad tried to chase the silliness of their tears away by mechanically slapping his son's back. Fran just tried to pull Walter closer to her, registering in her mind, but not on her face, the foreign, metallic stink of her son's breath.

The vacation sped by in a whirlwind of shopping trips, Christmas Eve, Christmas Day, exhausting rounds of visits to relatives . . . as usual. All three of them seemed to be operating on autopilot. They had performed these rituals in precisely the same way for years, and it gave them pleasure, exhilarated them, and wore them out. So dedicated was Fran to the celebration, to having her son home at last, that when the letters had come from the college, she put them up with the bills, unopened. Walter seemed fine, now that he was home. He smiled a lot, had a great time with his cousins, and when his favorite aunt and uncle, Elaine and Jack, asked him how his freshman year was going he nodded in a serious, almost embarrassed, boyish way and said he was having a grand time, though the work was "real tough."

Fran sensed there was more. She had felt something off-key in his letters home. His handwriting had deteriorated over the course of the semester. In September she could read his boyish but neat script with ease. By October, when he had sent her a bright purple leaf, the lines of his writing were no longer perfectly parallel. Some of them almost intersected. She received only one letter in November (after getting five in October), but the handwriting was hardly recognizable as Walter's. The individual letters were all different sizes, and the words they tried to form were poorly aligned. The ragged lines of words and thoughts seemed to loosen and fly off into nonsensical directions. The last third of the letter was impossible to read.

Fran had passed this off as the result of all the pressure Walter was under at school. His early letters had said it was nothing like high school, which had been a breeze for his sharp intelligence. His teachers had been in awe of the boy; many felt intellectually inferior to the brilliance of his gift. But from college her son had written her, "The teachers don't give a damn about me or what I have to say. They're too busy with their own research. All they want to hear from us is the exact same thing they said in their lectures. One of them wears the same tie every single day. My math teacher doesn't speak English—and none of us speak Korean!!!!!!! I guess I won't major in math!!!!!!!!!" Fran had chosen to interpret the exclamation points as signs of humorous exasperation.

When there was barely a week left in the vacation, Fran knew she would have to open the envelopes from the college, and chided herself for harboring such a silly foreboding. Walter never seemed to talk about college. When she had asked him if he made any friends there, his face had darkened and he turned away and mumbled, "A couple here and there."

"What about your roommate?"

"My roommate moved out." With that, Walter walked away from his mother.

[2]

With only six days before Walter's scheduled return to school, Fran took the packet of envelopes down from the shelf. Walter and his father were on an outing. Brad had taken a week's vacation from work to spend more time with his son. They would not return for hours, so Fran decided to lessen the importance of the envelopes from the college by opening and paying the household bills first. Electricity. Gas. MasterCard. Visa. Mortgage (only twelve more years to go: they had moved to this house the very week Walter started first grade. How he had cried when he had to leave Scruffy, the little mutt Brad had brought him that summer, and get on the bus, school bound). City tax installment. County tax installment. Water bill.

One of the envelopes from the college was shorter and narrower than a regular business envelope. It was the kind the credit card companies sent when you were behind in a payment. Maybe that's why it scared her, Fran thought. The other was a regular-size envelope. For some reason this one was even more ominous. It was from the dean's office, and their address had been personally typed, not printed by a computer like on the other.

Fran slipped her thumbnail under the edge of the small envelope and tore it open. It was a computer form: Walter's grades.

Math: F.

"How do they expect a boy to pass a course when it's not taught in English," Fran complained out loud, and made up her mind to write a letter to the university.

But though her attempt at indignation stirred her somewhat, the agitation failed to overcome a sense of falling, that some basic structure in her life, her son's intellectual indomitability, had broken down and was in the process of being swept away. Walter had never received a mark lower than a B since first grade, and precious few of those.

American history: F.

The blood inside Fran's heart pooled and turned to hot lead. Then it cooled and she hardened inside when she read that Walter received an F in literature, too.

She seemed to remember that her son had also taken chemistry. He loved chemistry, and had actually taken college-level chemistry at a local state college after exhausting his high school's chemistry courses. Fran found "Chemistry 100," but where the grade should have been there was only an I. This confused her, until she found the key and learned that it meant incomplete.

She collected herself and opened the other, larger envelope very carefully. But she found that her eyes couldn't proceed across the page in an orderly fashion. They just wanted to dance around the word "probation." She forced herself to read the letter over and over again until she understood that Walter could go back to school, but he had to pass all his courses, or that was it.

Then she read and understood the last few lines, "The college has an excellent counseling program for students experiencing difficulty adjusting to college life and pressures. May we advise that this service is available to Walter. . . ."

"Oh, Walter, baby," she whispered, and punctuated it by biting her lower lip. Fran was so frazzled that she gathered up all the envelopes and scraps, including her household bills, crumpled them until her hands were sweaty, and stuffed them into the trash can, pushing them down past the Christmas cards and coffee grounds.

That night she told Brad and said they should talk to Walter as soon as possible. Brad looked concerned, nodded gravely, frowned, said, "Of course," and then turned over and went to sleep, leaving Fran to wonder what she was going to say to her son. Walter was not the easiest person to talk to about difficult things. Fran and Brad had always known this. He was easily agitated—of course, he was so intense. His mind was a rocket ship, after all. And his fuse was short.

The next day, at the end of supper, Fran began casually, "Well, you'll be going back to school in a few days."

Walter looked at her as if she had slapped him awake, then got up from the table and began to pace back and forth, slipping his fingers over the wooden ridge atop the back of the chair as he passed by.

Brad said, in as conciliatory a tone as possible, "So, you didn't do so well this semester, eh?"

Walter stopped short, stared at his father, and asked, "What do you mean?"

Fran explained about the grade reports. Walter listened as a judge might cock his head to receive the alibi of an accused criminal— then waved it all away with a broad flourish. "It's just some goddamn computer error. I aced all those courses!"

Haltingly, Fran mentioned the letter from the dean.

Walter nodded, "Hmmmph! That old cracker doesn't know what's going on. He does what the computer tells him to do. Why, one year, the entire freshman class got those letters—all hand signed!"

Fran looked at her husband. It was time for a sigh of relief, but neither of them had the breath. Walter causally walked away, up to his bedroom.

Well, they'd had these kinds of scenes before.

Later, after Fran and Brad went to bed, Fran heard Walter tuning his guitar—at least that's what it sounded like at first, as the strings were struck loudly, deliberately, repetitively, one at a time. He hadn't played at all during the entire vacation. Fran had meant to ask him to play something, but there had been so much to do. The guitar had been his best friend all during his school years. He had taken lessons for more than seven years, and had become quite an accomplished player. For a while, he had his own rock-and-roll band. Fran said the music made her want to lose her sense of hearing, but she knew Walter understood she was only joking and that she was really very proud of the way his fingers flew nimbly over the strings and produced music clear and fine, rock-and-roll or not.

But that night something was wrong. Perhaps the inner structure of the guitar had been somehow damaged so that it could no longer play in tune, because Walter could not seem to progress beyond plucking the same note, an open string, seven or eight times before proceeding to the next string and doing the same. And over and over again.

Then he began plucking the notes randomly, and there were muffled, misbegotten notes that died in loud buzzes. There was no recognizable melody, only a jumble. Fran waited for the notes to arrange themselves, waited for her son to stop torturing her with this cacophony, waited for the beautiful music he had serenaded her with so many times as she had fallen off to sleep. It was not to come.

Well, he was angry at her and was punishing the guitar. Fran sensed that to believe otherwise would be to tip herself off the edge into despair.

[3]

The next three days passed as most of the vacation had. As the cycle was almost complete, the train station and the hugs and tears came into view again.

And then there was that last fine, pure morning of Fran's life, that last clean sky, that last day she could awaken, fill herself with a deep breath and let it out with a grateful smile. On that morning, she was coaxed out of her fuzzy first consciousness by the sound of a dog barking on the lawn just below her window. She recognized something painful in the sound of this animal that made her sick to her stomach. Trying not to wake Brad, she sat up in bed and leaned toward the window trying to see what was happening down on the lawn.

She could see nothing.

"Scruffy, I hear you, boy!"

Fran started to cry when she heard her son's voice speaking to a dog that had been dead for five years.

Walter spit out the words as if they were bitter pills, "I know you can understand people talk, Scruffy, but I think it would be a great idea if I could talk to you in dog language."

Fran's sobs shook harder when the barking started again. Walter came into view pacing ten feet below her second-story window. He was naked but for a pair of clumsy yellow galoshes.

"I won't let 'em take us back, Scruff, don't worry."

Fran shuddered. Her sobs became uncontrollable when Walter lay down on the lawn and she saw how wildly his eyes darted around as his head twitched defensively from side to side. Suddenly he jerked over on his side and huddled into a tense fetal crouch, shivering.

Fran was sobbing so violently by now that she had to draw in breath with a wail to keep from choking. She started pounding at Brad's still form under the blankets, to roust him to go down and get their son off the lawn.

It took Fran hours to regain her own grip on the minute-to-minute demands of consciousness. There was the agonizing visit by the police, who had responded to a call from a neighbor—a neighbor Fran would not be able to look in the eye for six years. The police did not insist on talking to Walter, but the boy walked out of the downstairs bathroom with a large bath towel wrapped around himself and proceeded to explain to them that they should do something about all the "real criminals in this world, and the evil men who assassinated Martin Luther King and President Kennedy and Pope John and Elvis who are hiding out right now at that college my mother wants me to go back to."

The police sergeant took Fran aside and told her that they could take Walter to the station, and that he would wind up at the county mental health center, "But if the family wants to make private arrangements. . ." Fran was shocked and felt coerced, but nevertheless picked up the phone in front of the policeman and made an emergency appointment with the family doctor, an internist, who agreed to see them later that day.

After the police left, Brad suggested they see Father Mooney, the pastor of their church. They went before lunch. Walter had calmed down enough to agree to accompany them. In fact, though his enormous tension was visible in the way his eyes kept darting around defensively and his hands never stopped clutching or rubbing or pounding his thighs, he looked the priest straight in the eye and told him that the pressures at college were enormous, but he thought he could make it. "It's a godless place, Father. I hate it."

Father Mooney seemed to be made extremely uncomfortable by the meeting, and when Walter took his hand and promised to do better, the aging priest seemed relieved. As he was ushering the family out the door, he held Brad back and whispered that he thought they were doing the right thing letting Dr. Howard see the boy.

Dr. Howard saw Walter first with Fran and Brad present, then alone. Though she couldn't pick out many specific words through the door, Fran could hear Walter's voice in long, energetic streams punctuated only by the low, brief hum of the physician's questions.

Then Dr. Howard asked to speak to Fran and Brad alone. He told them he thought Walter should see an "old friend" of his, Dr. Whitney. "Whit will be able to tell you how to help the boy. He'll have some suggestions."

"What's wrong with our boy?" Brad asked.

Dr. Howard raised his eyebrows. "I'm just a blood and guts man, you know that, Brad. The boy's in fine shape, as far as I can tell. He's lost a little weight, but they always go one way or the other their first year of college. But . . . my territory stops at his neck."

Fran and Brad stared at the doctor, not understanding.

"I mean . . . I'm really not the person to tell you what's going on in his head. Whit will do that. He's a fine physician."

That first visit to the psychiatrist was part of the blur now, a blur that in Fran's mind led back through the present darkness to a time when there was still hope, a feeling that she now equated with ignorance. People "hoped" when they believed their lives could still be put back together and recognized as their lives. Fran and Brad had left that point behind long ago, and were now struggling simply to survive in what was a grotesque caricature of their lives. That blur was a mix of countless visits to Dr. Whitney, who said he thought Walter might need some time in a private clinic, but that "We'll see."

And they had seen: four more breakdowns. Even living at home and taking classes at the nearby state college did not afford Walter more than a few months at a time of stability. Those early breakdowns had occurred at home. But then, as Fran had always feared, Walter "went public." One day he began pacing back and forth through the flow of sidewalk traffic, muttering his half of a conversation with Scruffy and spitting out bursts of incoherent criticisms of college life. A policeman came up just as Walter was unbuckling his belt.

Fran received a call from the county mental health center, which, she learned, was supposed to be a kind of "psychiatric emergency room" and outpatient clinic. She would learn a lot more about the place, as Walter found himself there too many times to count.

Then the blur intensified. Fran thought the blurring of memory might be a mental defense to insulate herself from the exquisite pain of every distinct moment. But the blur failed to do that as the pain intensified, too, with round after round of breakdown, private psychiatrist, private hospital, home, and then trips to inspect other facilities. Each had its own unique way of promising the same thing—a return to that infinitely simple universe where minds were vessels of the soul and worked in a partnership with each other and the world, not as combatants in a cruel and vindictive war of attrition. Each also had its own unique disappointment, as did the four-hundred-mile drive to talk to a maverick psychiatrist who promised to be able to get Walter back at the university with straight A's within a year. Fran and the doctor had gotten into a fight when the man had asked Walter, right in front of his parents, if he wanted to go to bed with his mother. She pulled Brad and Walter away and into the car.

The county clinic. The police. Dr. Whitney. Home. The allergist. The police. The neurosurgeon. The chiropractor-nutritionist. The county clinic again. A chance at the waiting list for an experimental program at the National Institute of Mental Health. The herbalist. The county clinic. Home. Jail.

[4]

Now, this bright winter morning ten years into Walter's illness, Fran wondered if there was any escape, if there was a place where she and her family could find sanctuary, a border beyond which this plague could not pursue them.

There was none. There was no place to go. They had run out of savings, and their private insurance had been canceled after Walter's fourth breakdown. The county clinic had suggested that it could do no more for Walter.

So they had come to the dreaded end of the line, the place where the blur solidified and in the sharp light of morning things became only too clear. The only place left was Bedloe State Hospital.

Fran had heard the mammoth upstate hospital described by people at the county center and at the private hospitals. When they had their guard down and didn't realize they were speaking in the presence of someone whose child might someday be sent there, they spoke about it the way the nuns in Fran's grammar school had described hell, casually using a word that was an unfortunate play on the name of the valley that gave its name and two thousand acres to the sprawling mental hospital.

Today Fran and Brad were driving their son to Bedlam.

2

Alex Greco, M.D., medical director of Bedloe State Hospital, was tensing in his sleep. His wife Maria could feel the quaking and knew he must be having his dream again. The quaking was a signal that he would soon wake up. She watched the beads of sweat sprout like crystal seedlings on his brow. His graying curly hair was already dark and flat with moisture.

Suddenly he was still, and letting go of a long, deep breath. Alex was awake.

Maria's voice was soft and caring, "You had the dream?"

"Yes, Maria, I had the dream again," Alex said with a touch of exasperation. He noted his own impatient tone and wondered whether he was impatient with his wife or whether he was actually impatient with his own unconscious for sending forth, as it had dozens of times over the past year and a half, the images that made waking up a rebirth into a soul-numbing pain that left him soaked, near-trembling, and weak on his back, staring up at the ceiling.

Maria embraced him across his chest.

"Maybe it had something to do with the call from Carmen."

Alex winced as if her statement was a blow to the same deep vulnerability that was already wounded and smarting.

"Yeah." He stirred and started to get up from beneath her embrace. "I guess," he sighed, sitting up on the other side of the bed from her. Maria's hand slipped down his back as he got up. He stood straight, inhaled deeply, and disappeared into the bathroom.

Twenty minutes later Alex emerged, fully dressed in his wool slacks and tweed sports jacket, complete with his red-and-blue school tie—seeming to stand taller by several inches than when he had arisen from bed. There was a forced smile on his face, but it signaled he was in control, that his depression was not going to weaken him. "The Doctor is here! Strike up the band!" he announced.

[2]

Alex self-consciously turned the key in the ignition of his well-preserved '69 Lincoln. The engine turned, whined, sputtered, and failed to start. Alex knew Maria was watching from the kitchen window. Though he knew his lines and stage positions well, it was always a struggle for him to keep his emotions to himself. Maria was an expert at seeing right through all his attempts to appear earnest and professional through his oatmeal and tea. Try as he might, it was usually impossible for him to get out of the house without showing her signs of the turbulence in his guts.

But this morning the slow, congestive churning didn't seem to be there. In the absence of the physical dread he'd felt so often lately, his smile felt more real. Alex knew that once he arrived at the hospital he would be transformed into the Physician and his bowels would get as close to stone still as they ever did.

Alex was not afraid or ashamed that his wife regularly saw through his mask. She knew everything about him, anyway. "Maria's a strong one," he was fond as saying. But this is my battle, he reasoned with himself. It was the jarhead in him. He hadn't spent those four years in the Marine Corps for nothing.

The Lincoln engine caught, and Alex backed out through a cloud of steam and exhaust.

Back at the window, Maria stood watching long after Alex had driven away. There was a quality of youth in the house, in the brightness of the colors and in the easy way the light filled the space. Maria applied herself crisply and with enthusiasm to every chore, every change, every challenge to the family's equilibrium—whether it was a problem one of the children had or Alex's emotional battles.

She shook her head and smiled—but then chased the pride away as an unfit emotion. Maria Greco was proud of that quality of youthful wildness and vulnerability in her husband. Most physicians she knew who were her husband's age, fifty-one, had long ago learned to give the appearance that they had everything under control in their lives. Alex had never tamed his adolescent wildness. He had very little under control, in the spiritual sense. He was always gentle, tender, and polite, yet his fury was always just a thin layer of civility away. His eyes could be as soft as a June sky or they could burn with a ferocious blue fire. The man had the ability to make clothes tailored just for him appear as though they had been hastily snatched off the rack at the local discount barn. It wasn't merely his six-foot body, which had the stocky, low-to-the-ground architecture of a warrior. It was the way his scrappy, stubborn nature did regular public battle with adversaries inside and out. There was nothing Alex could hide, either from himself or from those around him.

So Maria knew Alex thought he was going to get through the ride to the hospital this morning without the worms dancing around inside him.

As the big Lincoln cruised through town, Alex looked around at the village covered in last night's snow. The sky was deep blue, which made the snow all the more lustrous in the bright morning light. We were lucky, Alex mused. It was warmer than usual for January, despite the snow. Maybe it was time for the January thaw, when the temperature could rocket from the standard teens and twenties all the way up to the mid-sixties for a few days, sometimes for as long as a full week before plummeting.

The road was black and wet. He would have an easy ride. This time they would not need snowplows—but it was early. The Christmas decorations, not yet taken down from the village's five blocks of street lamps, seemed limp, somewhat shrunken, and embarrassed.

Thank God that season is past. Alex shook his head and drummed on the steering wheel with his finger. Now there would be a respite from the epidemic of suicide attempts at the hospital. The next epidemic would come as predictably as the movement of the planets, at the next equinox: spring.

Beyond the village the snow was deeper, but still not a problem. Alex felt safe nudging his Lincoln up to sixty. The road here was still a shiny wet black, not the dull matte that signals icy conditions. The big car needed the momentum to get up the mountain. Alex did not want to have to accelerate at the top where the snow was likely to be deeper because of the altitude, and where parts of the road sheltered by the woods from the morning sun might still be slushy. The top was a very dangerous spot, even under the driest, warmest conditions, because this was where the hospital first came into view.

Funny it should be that way. From that distance the hospital was a beautiful sight. And that was why the crest of the hill was such a dangerous spot. There was a highway turnoff built there especially for the view of the hospital. The legend was that the state highway department was obliged to build it because of the mounting death toll among tourists who were so distracted by the sudden dramatic view that they totally forgot what they were doing and either crashed through the railing into the gorge or plowed through groups of other tourists who had stopped to look or take photographs.

As was the custom at such viewing areas the department had installed a plaque: "Bedloe State Hospital. Built in 1913 to care for the mentally ill of the entire state. It is among the ten largest mental hospitals in the world." The county fathers had vigorously opposed the plaque. Let the tourists continue to think it was a castle, or a college. Many people mistook it for the local community college, which was twenty miles away and resembled a collection of army barracks.

In fact, the hospital's architects had envisioned a great European university. Alex smirked and wondered, as everyone connected with the hospital did, whether they had meant it as some kind of cruel joke, or whether the design was an expression of some genuine early twentieth-century enthusiasm and hope. In any case, the design, along with most jokes, enthusiasms, and hopes, was now an artifact.

Alex knew there would be a moment near the summit when the car would conquer the incline, stop straining against gravity, and seem, for a brief few moments, to lurch into flight. At that moment, the hospital would come into view. There were mornings when Alex closed his eyes for those few brief seconds, though the car was easily doing sixty-five. But even then he could still see the hospital, rising like a fortress, spreading itself over the land. The state had been generous and given more than two thousand acres for the site. They had envisioned a walled city and had built towers and parapets of stone.

The hospital was indeed a small city: one thousand patients and over two thousand staff members, including psychiatrists, psych techs, psychologists, nurses, social workers, psych interns, teachers, therapists, hospital workers, fire personnel, police, carpenters, and janitors. Bedloe had its own post office, fire department, canteen, pharmacy, beauty parlor, and medical-surgical infirmary. There were hospital wards for children, adolescents, and adults. There were forensic units for the mentally ill who had committed crimes, a unit for patients who were mentally retarded as well as mentally ill, a unit for the hearing-impaired, a unit for neurologically im-paired victims of trauma, a geriatric unit, and special security units for violent patients.

Suddenly, as the viewing area came up, Alex slowed the Lincoln and turned so abruptly that the tires screeched as he pulled off the road into the shallow parking lot. The car skidded a bit on the fresh snow, but tore through to the gravel and came to a stop. Alex got out of the car and walked past the end of the wall and over to the edge of the hill, where the unobstructed view crawled right up the mountain to his feet.

This morning the main tower, which was over two hundred feet tall, seemed to rise out of the mist that blanketed the lower floors of the building. And there were the lesser towers of the fire house, the kitchen, and the steeple of the chapel. The sun was already starting to burn off the mist, so the ghostly forms of the buildings were beginning to materialize, as were the parapets of the Great Wall, which slinked over hill and dale like a giant stone reptile.

The wall was originally intended to encircle the entire hospital grounds. But the ambitiousness of the state legislature ran out long before the hundreds of acres of woods beyond the buildings. You couldn't see the exact spot from here, but the elaborate stonework of the wall abruptly gave way to a ten-foot-high wire fence some- where amidst the trees. But even that failed to complete the state's attempt to establish a boundary. There were large gaps in the fence, and places so wild and thick with forest that they had never even been adequately surveyed, let alone fenced.

But from this comfortable distance the human eye could take it all in. That's why Alex often stopped here before descending into Bedloe Valley. There was something at Bedloe that got to Alex, something elemental, a raw and primitive force that burrowed its way into him and built a lair in the midst of his most vulnerable tissues.

He took in a long, deep breath of the crisp air of the New Year. The damp air of the valley coiled up at his feet, and Alex shuddered in the chill.

[3]

A sheet of snow clouds snuck into the valley as Alex approached the hospital. Large, clumsy snowflakes landed heavily on his wind- shield. There was nothing ominous at all about the hospital en- trance. The stonework at the front gate was beautiful. Alex saw why it could be mistaken for a college campus even at this proximity: Here were landscaped grounds with tall attractive trees; here were people walking casually between neatly arranged buildings, some a bit more deliberate, no doubt intent on making it to class with the morning's cramming intact.

It was only when you came a little closer that something didn't quite fit. There were discordant notes here, rhythms out of sync, some subtly, some grotesquely. You didn't see it, yet you sensed it, the grotesquerie was in the spirit of things. There was a presence here, a joker tripping the gods who conceived and gave birth to each successive moment. In this universe the planets lurched and bumped through space.

Now Alex could see a man walking as if his right leg had to be dragged, but every third step was perfectly normal. There was a woman standing with her face upturned to the gray sky, who didn't even blink when the snowflakes came to rest in her eyes.

And here came a squad of children walking in such a perfect line they seemed to be tethered to each other like sled dogs trudging through the snow—and not one of them broke away to play in it, not one of them as much as stooped to grab a handful of it. They didn't even notice it. As they passed a fenced-in yard, a man watched them from the other side of the wire. His eyes were vacant of everything but his hunger, yet his face was calmly smiling at some inevitability he alone was aware of. At the top of his fence the coils of razor-wire glistened like new tinsel.

From one of the buildings there came sounds of plates clattering and breaking, pots and pans ringing, knives and forks jousting, and the smells of burnt meat and toast. Alex sensed the pouring of milk under bright lights and the hoarding of sugar in dusty closets.

The windows glowed. There was life behind them, figures moving, some slowly, some abruptly, some standing still, perhaps watching. Voices . . . chanting, mixed with the sorrowful snowfall. Then he began to feel the band tightening inside, the desire to flee.

Alex fought his sense of dread and kept on walking toward his office. There will be spring days when the sun is bright and there are flowers all around this place, he reminded himself. The snow could barely hide the fact that the grounds were exquisitely landscaped.

On the steps of the main building, Alex paused for an old man being led as if he were blind. But he was not blind. He looked right at Alex and saw him and said to him, "I'm just fine, you know. They won't let me tell anybody." He paused to gather his words and rolled his tongue around his mouth as if the letters were marbles that had to be assembled before they could be spoken. "I don't belong here. I don't belong here!" Then his face opened like a child's. "This is a bad place." He fell silent and the black man helping him across the yard smiled kindly and helped him up the steps.

Alex made a point to arrive early every morning, before most of the day-shift physicians and staff. He entered his office, and the phone was already ringing. It was Wendy Dixon, a psych tech who usually worked in another ward, calling him from the Receiving Unit, where she was filling in. The police had brought in an attempted suicide and Wendy could not find a psychiatrist to come down. She had seen his car enter the hospital grounds. Alex knew there were plenty of psychiatrists on duty around the hospital, but he was grateful because it gave him the opportunity to do some clinical work. Though Alex was the medical administrator and, therefore, responsible for every patient in the hospital, except for occasional and brief sessions most of his contact with patients was via paperwork. Some administrative physicians liked it that way; in fact, they got into administration just so they would not have to deal with patients eye-to-eye. Not Alex.

Wendy told him she would meet him halfway with the chart.

"Huh? Why?"

"The parents are here, Doctor."

"Oh, Christ! Parents! It's a kid?"

"A nineteen-year-old girl."

Alex's rib cage tightened. A kid. If there was anything he dreaded more than crazy kids, it was suicidal kids. When things got rough, he tended to lose it as a physician and start acting like a father.

The thought crossed his mind to ask Wendy if there was anyone else who could handle this, but he held back on the impulse. That would be desertion of duty under fire. In the Corps they shot guys for that. Alex stripped off his jacket and pulled on his white coat. He was out the door in a flash, but then he ducked back in to grab his stethoscope.

As promised, Wendy met him halfway with the chart. Alex thought of her as a handsome woman. She was too big-boned and powerful looking to be called pretty. Besides, Wendy would have socked anyone who called her that.

Lily Speere had scrawled a note to her parents that she had "swallowed a bottle of pills." They weren't quite sure yet what kind of pills—Lily had hidden the empty bottle. Her stomach had been pumped and blood tests and stomach-contents tests were underway and would be completed soon.

"Any nausea?"

"Yes, Doctor."

"Won't she talk, Wendy?"

"Nope. Her lips are sealed."

"Parents deny drug abuse," Alex noted out loud from the chart, seeking Wendy's confirmation, fishing for details about them before actually asking her.

"They deny everything," Wendy said with a smirk and a shrug.

They rounded the corner and Alex scanned the loosely arranged red chairs in the wide hallway, which was the unofficial waiting room for the Receiving Unit. The unit was officially for receiving new patients transferred from other facilities, not for drive-in psychiatric emergencies. But since the nearest county hospital with a psychiatric unit was more than forty-five miles away, Bedloe tended to get a lot of walk-in, or drive-in, emergencies. How did you tell a local population of almost 100,000 people and a police and emergency force of several hundred that they were not supposed to send mentally ill patients to this gigantic mental hospital where a hundred psychiatrists were sitting around on their hands?

So Bedloe got emergency psychiatric cases. One of the largest mental hospitals in the United States, and perhaps the world, also doubled as a psychiatric field hospital.

Alex saw no one out of place in the hall, no people who could be the girl's parents.

"Wendy, where are Mom and Dad?"

"Uhhh . . . in with their daughter."

"Christ!"

This was going to be rougher than Alex had imagined.

"Okay, where is she?"

"Right there, 105."

The door was ajar, and even before he looked in, Alex could hear a low, cadenced murmur, as if a priest were saying last rites. He knew that couldn't be, not yet, since the chart said the girl's vital signs were all good. Of course, it wouldn't be the first time a chart was botched.

"O this is the poison of deep grief. . . ."

It wasn't a priest. It was a small, balding man in a tweed jacket sitting beside the bed, hunched over the still form, staring right at her as he recited, "When sorrows come, they come not single spies but in battalions. . . ."

Alex had heard those words before. The rhythm was familiar, and when he recognized the author, his mouth dropped open. Holy Mother! he thought. The man is reciting Shakespeare!

"Poor Ophelia, divided from herself and her fair judgment, without the which we are pictures, or mere beasts. . . ."

In the corner, sitting in a red vinyl chair, the mother stared at her daughter's face as if this were the girl's only link with this world and she was not about to let go. And the girl's face . . . was so calm and gentle. Her features were delicate, a saint in repose.

Alex took a deep breath, pushed the door open, and walked in. "Hello, I'm Doctor Greco. Mrs. and Mrs. Speere?"

The mother started to rise, but the father just fell silent and kept staring at his daughter. Alex ignored him and turned his attention to the mother, who was now standing. The two of them looked at the father, who did not acknowledge either of them. Alex realized that the guy was in complete control of the room, which was exactly the way he no doubt wanted it. Alex started wishing there had been a monster snowstorm—then he would have been half an hour late, at least.

Alex looked at Lily again. Her eyes were closed. She was perfectly still. Not acknowledging Alex, the father stood up, and then, finally, turned.

"I'm Dr. Greco." Alex held out his hand.

"Dr. Edward Speere."

Alex looked the man over. He didn't look like a physician.

"Professor of comparative literature at Tri-C."

Alex inwardly breathed a sigh of relief.

"When can we take Lily home, Doctor?" the mother asked.

"Well . . . I don't exactly know, Mom. I want to get some information from you and Dad, here. I want to find out what happened . . . and all that . . . and . . ." Alex started to usher them out of the room.

"Nothing happened. Nothing happened at all," the mother said. She's very high strung. And—"

"Excuse me, Joan," the father cut in. "Something obviously happened, otherwise she wouldn't be lying here in this hospital. The girl tried to do herself in. And she did it to get at us."

"Let's go in the hallway, folks, please," Alex tried to insist.

But it was too late. Alex was aware of a slight stirring on the bed— just enough movement for the expansion of the chest to allow air in, or perhaps a mild gasp . . . and then, booming, "I G-G-G-GO F-F-

F-FORTH TO C-C-C-C-C-CREATE THE UNCREATED C-C-C-C-CONSCIOUSNESS OF M-M-M-MY RACE!"

Alex sensed the parents' alarm and bore down on them, "You folks are going to have to leave right now—Wendy!"

Wendy was a more than even match for the parents. She came in with a confident smile and her arms already outstretched in a herding gesture. "Okay, Mom and Dad, we need to let the doctor do his work here. I have to get some information from you, just step outside here, please." This was no request: Wendy didn't leave them any choice. There was not the least hesitation in her step: They either went her way or resisted her physically. So in one fluid movement, the parents were swept out of the room and Alex was alone with Lily . . . who was lying flat. Only now her eyes were open and burning with the terror of a small animal caught in a huge trap. Those huge blue eyes met Alex's and he went tight inside, protecting himself against the melting he knew could happen if he let it.

"I f-f-eel sick," she murmured. The color drained from her face.

"Wendy!" Alex called, as he instinctively reached for the girl's wrist. Damn the state for not installing those buzzers he had requisitioned months ago. The girl's pulse was racing. "Wendy!"

"I f-f-feel real sick now. I'm going to throw up."

Lily started to sit up. Alex noted that her blond, silky hair had been unevenly hacked. Some patches were two feet long, some just an inch or so, most were somewhere in between. As the girl started to retch, Wendy was at her side with a pan. Alex knew he should turn away, but he was transfixed by the girl's face as the convulsions moved across her body as if she were driftwood atop a violent sea.

"Blood's okay," Wendy remarked, as Lily started to cough, "just mildly elevated salicylates."

That was the news Alex was waiting for. Whatever Lily had swallowed—apparently aspirin—had overwhelmed her stomach's ability to absorb it.

"The parents stabilized?"

Wendy nodded. "For now."

Alex took some tissues and wiped Lily's mouth. Then, with a clean cloth at the bedside, he gently wiped the sweat from her brow. "I think she's gonna be okay, Wendy. But let's not be hasty here."

"You bet, Doctor." and she was out of the room as effortlessly as she had appeared.

Alex looked at Lily and censored the "Well, young lady?" that was on his lips. Instead, he asked her, "How do you feel now?" After he said it, he realized it, too, was fatherly. He couldn't escape it: whatever he said came out like a parent.

"My stomach b-b-b-burns."

"Ummm hmmmm."

"And my soul b-b-burns, too," she frowned.

"I guess it does. You could have hurt yourself pretty bad."

The frown melted away, and she was a sweet little girl again. "I just t-took some aspirin, that's all."

"Why?"

"The M-m-mothers said it was a good thing."

"Your mother told you to do it?"

"No, not my m-mother—the M-m-m-m-mothers."

The conversation went on. Lily knew the time, the day, and the date, and she could accurately locate herself in the moment in the right town, right state, right country, right planet in the right solar system. That was something, anyway. More than two-thirds of the patients at the hospital couldn't.

But the child was disturbed: she had tried to hurt herself. Alex let her go on about the Mothers, who, Lily explained, were mythical characters who spoke to her through the volumes of poetry and folklore and science fiction she read—and who sometimes spoke to her directly when she, herself, wrote. Lily described the inspirational trances she would invoke, during which the lines she wrote "don't c-c-come from me at all, but from the M-m-mothers, who speak through my hand."

Alex took several deep breaths. He knew that in any major city, at that moment, there were dozens of people making a fine living selling other people the "collected wisdom" they matter-of-factly declared came not from them but from some kind or another of bodiless "entity."

But this wasn't a major city, this was Bedloe State Hospital, and this little girl had just tried to take her own life. Alex scraped away his parental instincts and allowed his diagnostic ones to assert themselves: the girl needed treatment. She needed to stay here, or somewhere. This might not be the best place, but there was nowhere else within a hundred miles that could even begin to help her. She needed constant observation because she meant business.

This was one time he was sure. Other docs might look for two or three or four or more signs before making a decision, whether or not they had the sense of what was going on—and most did have it. Only most didn't listen to it, didn't trust it.

Alex had learned to trust his. There were plenty of signs to point to, but he could feel it in the room, feel the tragedy and sickness.

The parents would be a big problem, Alex suspected. If the girl had broken her leg, there would be no question in their minds that she needed medical attention. They would fight for it if they had to. But although Lily was every bit as ill as if both her arms and legs had messy compound fractures, this was different. This was mental illness, and the entire process was still mired in fear, shame, and revulsion. As stubbornly as the parents would demand medical attention when they could see the blood and the broken flesh, they would now resist it, because the precise lesions in their daughter's substance were still beyond anyone's ability to detect, measure, and describe.

It would be far too much trouble to try to get the girl committed without their cooperation. They would have their lawyers in court within twenty-four hours, and they would do their best to make the doctor out to be a damn fool for trying to lock away their little girl in "that awful place."

Alex would try to convince them.

"Lily, I've enjoyed talking to you. Now, I'm going to talk to your parents, okay?"

She shrugged and looked away. The girl, Alex mused as he left the room, would be easy to convince to stay.

"Mom and Dad," Alex chose to address them informally, "I believe Lily needs some treatment. I think she should stay here."

"Absolutely not," the father declared.

Mrs. Speere just closed her eyes and shook her head.

"I think we were lucky this time, but next time she might make it and"—Alex choked on the words—"succeed in killing herself."

"Lily is not sick," the mother said. "She's high strung. Alienated— because of her intelligence and creativity—mind you. But she's not sick." This was said with sad conviction, almost resignation, as if she had gone over this time and time again, persuading herself that it was bad, but more acceptable than being "mentally ill."

Dr. Speere rose. "When can we take our daughter home, Doctor?"

Alex paused before speaking, and measured his opponents.

"It's really too premature for a full diagnosis, but your daughter is obviously in the throes of a major depressive episode. Her buoyancy is a surface quality, a mask. She has a tendency toward grandiose delusions—and she's flirting with psychosis. She's in a great deal of pain and needs to be helped."

"We'll take her to our family doctor. He'll refer us, if we need it," the father pronounced.

Alex couldn't stay to watch Lily's parents sign her out. Wendy came over and he let her handle the rest. As he turned away from the Speeres, he noticed a new group entering the Receiving Unit. A psych tech who usually accompanied new patients coming to Bedloe from a county across the state was ushering in a man who walked slowly, tentatively, meek and frightened as a four-year-old being led into the doctor's office for the first time. Yet the new patient had mostly gray hair and the face of a middle-aged man.

Alex knew that was no clue to his actual age. He could be in his twenties.

The new patient was hesitating in the doorway. "Walter, it's okay," the psych tech said. Behind the new patient an older man and woman came in the outer door. More parents, Alex could tell. The father, who was bald and wore wire-rim glasses, looked bent over, weary. Alex had seen fathers of the mentally ill acquire this posture: an almost ashamed meekness, a desire to disappear. The mother affected no such timidity. She stood straight and seemed taller than she actually was. Her hair was bright blond even to the point of appearing brassy, and her green eyes flashed with a deep fire.

She came up to her son's side and squeezed his hand between hers. "What is it, Walter?"

"What is this place?" the new patient murmured weakly.

By now other Receiving Unit staff were on the scene, so Alex decided to leave. The woman had not yet answered her son. She was looking around the unit as if trying to gather enough information or composure—and her eyes met Alex's.

Alex stood still. He would help if needed.

But the woman turned to her son and spoke softly, "It's the hospital we talked about, Walter. You know."

Released, Alex turned and left.

[4]

On the way back to his office, Alex tried to shove the experience
with the Speeres back into some vault of professional disappoint-
ments, the kind of place where surgeons buried the patients who
died. But there was no such place for Alex. He looked around him
and realized that he was *in* the place where other psychiatrists
buried the patients they had lost. Like Walter. Walter Channing, Alex
remembered his name from the file of incoming patients. Chronic
schizophrenia. Standard history: in and out of private and public
institutions. And now, finally, here.

Alex shook it off. Sure, some people might ask why Lily Speere's
parents should allow their daughter to be admitted to a place that
was a last resort, where people came when there was no other place
to go. Some might say that the girl's chances were better out of this
hospital than in it. But Alex couldn't really believe that. He knew her
chances were a shade brighter in the hospital. Alex had to have that
increment of light; it was his entire reason for continuing here.

He was angry at the girl's parents, but he knew it was the
psychiatrist in him who was angry. The parent in him was terrified
for the girl, just as they were. It wasn't their fault. Certainly there
might be some family problems that set the girl off one way or the
other, but chances were good there were brothers and sisters who
had grown up in the same family under the same circumstances and
turned out fine.

But the parents would be blamed anyway. Even psychiatrists who
were properly schooled in the latest research, those who knew and
understood that mental illness was a physical disease of the brain,
that Lily's intricate biological wiring was somehow malfunctioning
—even they would feel a tightening in the chest around the parents.
*You did this to your child. You made certain crucial mistakes at
critical times and now look. Look at the pain your child is in! You
gave her bad cereal, bad toilet training, bad schooling, bad genes!
You brought this pain into the world.*

As a parent and a psychiatrist, Alex knew that wasn't fair. But he
also knew that the game didn't start out fair. Why should it begin to

be fair in some late inning when the score was already lopsided against the kid?

But who could be blamed for this unfair horror? Alex asked himself over and over again.

[5]

Back in his office, Alex closed his eyes tightly and pinched his eyebrows together. His day was spread out before him in the paperwork on the desk. His secretary, who had arrived while Alex was at the Receiving Unit, had added to the pile. There were medical reports of one kind or another that had to be reviewed, new patient admissions, discharge papers to sign, reports of medical problems ranging from drug reactions to nonmental illnesses to injuries, minutes of administrative meetings to acknowledge, requests for meetings. . . . Maybe Doc Rush would show up, as he often did this time of day, before Alex had to plunge into it.

The walls of Alex's office were decorated with several paintings he had done himself, some copied from photographs or old pictures, depicting significant events in the history of care of the mentally ill. In the center of the wall opposite the desk was the largest of the paintings, in which a group of well-dressed men and women in eighteenth-century finery stood on a second-floor gallery and observed a large room below them crowded with what were then called "lunatics," who wore coarse gray linen clothes. Immediately below the spectators, three or four of the lunatics reached up in supplication. The observers smiled and blessed them with crusts of bread they pulled out of a sack. Other wretches groveled on the floor for crumbs. Many sat in darker corners of the room, staring. One woman appeared to be shaking her fist at the amused gentry.

When a psychiatrist or psychologist saw Alex's painting, invariably he or she would assume it was the infamous St. Mary's of Bethlehem Hospital in London, founded in 1247. Through the years, the hospital's name, slowly corrupted into Bedlam, had become synonymous with inhumane care of the mentally ill.

But Alex was quick to correct them: the painting was not a scene in London, but in eighteenth-century Philadelphia, where the first hospital in America to admit the mentally ill also admitted, temporarily, of course, and for a small fee, citizens of the city who wished to spend an hour or so entertained by the lunatics.

Only one person had not required Alex's correction. That was Doc. The seventy-two-year-old psychiatrist had walked into the office, looked at the canvas, nodded, and said, "Nice picture of Pennsylvania Hospital. . . . You know, my great-great-great-great-great-great-grand-uncle ran the place for a while."

Alex had taken to Doc immediately. In a hospital stocked with over a hundred physicians, Woodrow Benjamin Rush was the only one called Doc. He had earned the moniker. Doc was practicing psychiatry before most of the staff of Bedloe was potty-trained.

"Is this bar open for business?" It was Doc, poking his head through the doorway. He was a tall, gangly man, with a full head of white, shaggy hair which he wore in a long, almost foppish manner. His trademark red bow tie added to the effect.

"Happy New Year, Doc. C'mon in."

Alex had noticed something special in Doc the first time they met, as soon as he asked the routine question he posed to all psychiatrists under him: "Why did you become a psychiatrist?"

"My mother was enamored of a surgeon," Doc had begun. "And my Irish grandmother wanted me to be a priest—so I split the difference."

Alex read the sparkle in Doc's eye, and knew that here was a psychiatrist who earnestly loved the profession. Doc had demonstrated that love at the beginning of his career by trading his nonpsychiatric assignments for his fellow students' psychiatric ones. After a distinguished thirty-year-plus career, Doc had retired—but only from private practice, not from psychiatry. He was now the psychiatrist in Wilson Cottage, a co-ed unit of severely ill patients.

Alex looked forward to any time he could spend with Doc. Since Doc had lived through all the upheavals in psychiatry of the last half-century, he was able to comment on them with a sense of history that comforted Alex, who was forced by the responsibilities of his job and the tendencies of his personality to give too much weight to the present and immediate future.

Now, Alex's eyes were drawn to the patient file Doc was carrying.

"You really are here on business."

"Well . . . it's Greta Lampson."

Alex nodded. "Refractory depression."

"I knew you wouldn't need to see the file." A brief smile and a nod of admiration played across the left side of Doc's face.

Alex remembered the important details of just about every patient in the hospital. "It's my job to know what's going on here with the patients."

"Sure it is." Doc sat down and tucked the unneeded file between his hip and the plush arm of the chair. "But you're the first medical director I've ever seen who not only takes that part seriously but who actually can do it."

Alex deflected the praise. "She's in a bad way."

Doc took a candy bar out of his jacket pocket and started to unwrap it. "The woman is so suicidal, we may have to invent a new diagnosis. She's determined to die. She has a whole mythology built around doing herself in." Doc offered Alex the opportunity to decline the chocolate bar before taking a bite himself.

"Maybe it goes with the hormones," Alex said. "Women romanticize their depression. They hear the music. Play it in their minds as they're swallowing the pills or slitting their wrists. The poetry of death."

"I've had male patients who've done that, too."

"So have I, but they tend to be men with a lot of the feminine anima to begin with."

"You're right," Doc jumped in. "Women are devilishly clever about it. They can put an incredible amount of energy into articulating their depression as a romantic story. Sometimes you don't even know they're depressed until you find them dead."

"So . . . Greta Lampson. I think I know why you're here."

Alex knew, and dreaded the discussion. First, because he knew it involved bureaucratic procedures, second, because Doc's scorn for bureaucratic protocol was legendary, and third, because it would be Alex's responsibility to enforce the rules.

Doc nodded solemnly, chewing on the last of the chocolate.

"You've tried everything else?"

Doc kept nodding.

"At least three months' trial with each drug?"

"Anybody who needs three months to tell if a medication is

working on depression should consider, perhaps, becoming a chiropractor." Doc's impatience with the process was breaking through.

"I know that—but the lawyers are in charge here, and they say you've got to go through a three-month trial with every antidepressant known to man before you can even think about ECT."

"Don't forget," Doc said, "I was one of the psychiatrists who testified against that silly rule when the legislature took it up. Sometimes electroconvulsive therapy is the only thing that works, I told 'em!"

"And it is," Alex nodded. "And it is."

"ECT has saved lots of lives. I think it can save Greta. I'll sign the papers."

"You'll have to go to court."

"Gladly."

"Most physicians avoid it."

"One of my nephews is a judge. I guess every judge has had his diapers changed at one time in his life. They don't scare me."

"Okay, Doc. We'll begin the paperwork."

"Thanks, Alex. I want to save this patient."

"You want to save them all, Doc." Alex smiled, relieved that the discussion was over and Doc's sense of humor was still intact.

"That's not true. I know they all can't get well. But I know they can all get better. And that's what I'm here to do." Doc appeared to be staring at one of Alex's paintings. Alex recognized this as Doc's cue for a story.

"You know, we used to think of ECT as a godsend. It worked so well in the psych ward at City General that they almost had the bars removed from the windows. Imagine that! Before we had electroconvulsive therapy, we used a drug to induce the convulsions. As soon as you injected it, before the convulsions came on, the patient would give a big yawn. That was one of the problems with it. The yawn was so intense that a lot of people would dislocate their jaws."

Alex knew this was something he'd heard about or read in psychiatry texts, but by the time he was in training it had been ancient history.

"To keep them from biting their tongue, we'd wrap a wad of cotton and gauze into a tube and take it with both thumbs and stick it in the mouth between the teeth. Well, I was giving it to one patient and I wasn't fast enough and the convulsions started with both my hands in his mouth. I stood there until he finished his convulsions, praying I'd still have all my fingers."

Both men laughed. Thank God for Doc.

3

[1]

At the private psychiatric hospital in New England where Woodrow Rush was trained, many of his patients came from thousands of miles away. One woman rode up in a chauffeur-driven Rolls-Royce and entered the hospital with her own cook and servant. When he told that story, Doc always chuckled at the end, "A little different from our average patient here in the state hospital."

Doc had a patient there from Cedar Rapids, Iowa, whose general practitioner would visit her from home every couple of months. The end of his training happened to coincide with her discharge. Her physician came up to see him—they had had many talks over the two years she was his patient—and asked if he was interested in coming to Iowa to practice psychiatry. The GP said he had patients waiting for Doc. So the young psychiatrist went to Cedar Rapids. That was his first practice. Within a month he was chief of psychiatry at two local hospitals—by virtue of the fact that he was the only psychiatrist in town.

31

But the aroma of oats and the rolling prairie that made an island out of Cedar Rapids only made young Woodrow Rush restless. There was a big war going on, and he wanted to be a part of it—and sail on the real ocean. So Doc joined the Navy, which was only too happy to have him. The war's appetite for psychiatrists was insatiable. Since Doc already was one, the Navy put him in charge of training new ones. "If a physician admitted to walking past a state hospital during his lifetime, that was enough for us. He was immediately drafted into advanced training for psychiatry."

Telling this story, Doc always went silent for a long moment, savoring the memory. Then his eyes opened wider and he smiled. "Interestingly enough . . . quite a few of those people actually stayed in psychiatry and went for more training after the war."

"I trained some of them, too," Doc would say, with a proud twinkle in his eye. "I always try to show my appreciation for life's minor ironies."

It had been one of those ironies that brought Doc to Bedloe State Hospital—an irony whose seed had been planted and slowly germinated over the long course of Doc's career.

By the early 1950s, Doc was busily on his way to establishing one of the most distinguished private psychiatric practices in his hometown, a city of more than half a million people. Doc began as a psychoanalyst. The introduction of tranquilizing drugs did not slow him down. Although many analysts were derailed by a drug that promised to reduce psychotic symptoms in a matter of days, Doc greeted the drugs as just another potentially useful tool.

Although many analysts resisted the trend, Doc saw right away that the future of psychiatry was one that would include drugs. He knew more drugs would be invented and readily used by the new psychiatrists he was training. Furthermore, he found medications helped his severely ill patients.

Keeping up with the latest advances on all fronts, Doc also developed a more supportive, action-oriented psychotherapy. Because his personal psychotherapy was so effective—and so satisfying to him—he could never bring himself just to prescribe a drug and collect a fee. He felt he wasn't being a psychiatrist unless he did some psychotherapy. So Doc was one of the first psychiatrists to come to terms with the drug revolution by realizing that the best therapy combined both drugs and psychotherapy. Of course, as far as Doc was concerned, it was best because it made people happy all around: It made him happy because he got to do what he wanted to do, which was psychotherapy; it made the drug companies happy because they sold some drugs and could point to some improving patients; it made the patients happy because they felt they were getting the most modern treatment available—as well as getting to spend some time talking to the doctor. His patients liked spending time with him, no matter what the drugs promised or delivered.

So Doc's career went its merry way for thirty years. Then one day an article in a medical journal snagged his attention, a rare occurrence. This article happened to be a panel discussion on the role of psychotherapy in the treatment of severe mental illness. The way Doc described it, "Here were these three psychiatrists going around in circles on whether or not psychotherapy has a role. I couldn't make heads or tails out of any of their arguments, which made me feel as though a once happy part of my life was actually a failure—I had trained all three of those fellows."

Doc wrote a letter to the journal—not, of course, criticizing the three eminent physicians, but declaring that psychiatric drugs and psychotherapy had coexisted very nicely in his practice for thirty years and that the three of them—"the drugs, the therapy, and me"—had proved an effective partnership for his many patients.

It was the only letter Doc had ever written to a journal, so, naturally, he examined every forthcoming issue for it. Finally, five months later, his letter appeared. Everything was spelled correctly and the editors had not made a single change. But they had apparently allowed the original three psychiatrists to comment on Doc's letter. Only one took the opportunity. His reply appeared under Doc's letter: "Our panel was charged with discussing the relative merits of combined therapy in cases of severe mental illness. I am sure that in Dr. Rush's long and distinguished career, he has seen some of these. However, what is effective for the psychiatrist treating what some have referred to as 'the worried well' may not be so effective in the seriously ill patient. . . ."

Doc felt the words strike him like a powerful blow. He frowned and threw the magazine across the room. But later that evening he picked it up and started leafing through it, questioning his entire life as he did. He knew that many of his patients over the past thirty years had been seriously ill—had been, in fact, just about as mentally ill as a person could be. Others were, to be sure, the "worried well," people with fundamentally healthy personalities who were depressed or anxious or, as Doc liked to say, curious. Doc had, after all, begun his career at a time when psychiatrists were the primary helpers for people who wanted to explore their own minds, a time when psychiatrists were the priests who mediated between a human being and the powerful forces that flowed through the mind from God knows where.

Until the afternoon he read the response to his letter Doc had believed that his life and career contained the sweep of the entire profession, that as a psychiatrist Woodrow Benjamin Rush was complete as well as distinguished. But then, in his sixties, Doc was restless, and a restless man will doubt the value of the road he's taken, despite its grandeur, if he's got the itch for some different scenery. Doc had that itch, and so when he turned the page and his eyes happened to fall on the relatively tiny ad in the "Psychiatrists Wanted" section of the classifieds, the ad that read: "TIRED OF TREATING THE WORRIED WELL?" and then on the next line: "Call or write Alex Greco, M.D., Medical Director, Bedloe State Hospital," he knew for the first time how those ninety-day wonders during the war felt when he recruited them for psychiatry.

Doc, in writing the letter that answered Alex's ad, had all the youthful flush of a man who is going to the front and knows only the parades and the waving girls and the bright clean horizon of his life still reaching farther than he can see.

[2]

Bedloe was temporary home for a number of young physicians receiving their residency training at the hospital. After their time serving as quasi-apprentices to senior psychiatrists, they would move on to their final preparation for psychiatric practice. The time at the state hospital was meant to expose them to the most severely ill patients, which Bedloe had in abundance.

Alex Greco was in charge of distributing the residents among the psychiatrists. To Doc he had assigned one Steven Rose. From Rose's file, Alex knew that the young man was an excellent student and his previous teachers had vigorously recommended him for psychiatry. He was genuinely interested in the welfare of his patients, which would make him a good physician. Two references had commented that he sometimes seemed perhaps too interested.

His advisor had thought he might do well as a psychoanalyst, where he really wouldn't have to take aggressive medical responsibility for a patient's illness—at least not to the same extent as a psychiatrist administering psychoactive drugs or electroconvulsive therapy.

Since Doc had successfully made the transition from a plush, comfortable psychoanalyst's office to the linoleum-tiled state hospital wards, Alex figured if anyone could smoke the psychiatrist out of this kid, it was Doc.

Doc could tell in the early moments of their first meeting on the ward that his young charge, who looked about as much like a lost terrier as anyone could, was unable to tell the patients from the staff, except in cases where the staff person was wearing a badge or a uniform. Were it not for Rose's own white coat and stethoscope, the profound discomfort and disorientation he radiated might have allowed him to blend in with the patients fairly well. Though the resident had obviously assembled all the equipment necessary for a professionally neat appearance—tie, short haircut, well-tailored suit, wing-tips—Doc was aware of a certain dishonesty in the execution. His white coat was buttoned out of sequence, giving Dr. Rose a decidedly unbalanced bearing. "Well," Doc later told Alex during one of their frequent conversations, "I'm always saying that psychiatry teaches you patience. I'm eternally hopeful. Now's my chance to prove it."

Doc took most of the month of February just to introduce Dr. Rose to Wilson Cottage. He started with psych tech Wendy Dixon. As far as Doc was concerned, the psych techs were the front-line troops, the ones in the trenches. Doc acknowledged to Rose that a lot of physicians and other staff thought he was being too generous to the psych techs, but he also pointed out that the techs worked hands on with the patients more than anyone else in the hospital. He admitted that it was an exaggeration to say that a mental hospital could run without doctors if it simply had enough psych techs. But, as far as Doc was concerned, it was a minor exaggeration.

Besides, the only way Rose could become properly initiated into Wilson Cottage was through Wendy. Even before the young physician knew what Wilson Cottage was, he would have to know Wendy. Wendy was the chief psych tech in Wilson Cottage, a status conferred more from her genuine value and role than from any official title. The patients loved her, and with good reason. Wendy was their best friend. "She's dedicated," Doc told Rose: "More important, she's joyous about it. You get dedicated people who make a penance out of it, so it becomes a trial for everybody else, too. Wendy spends a lot of her own time and money on the patients—and that's not part of her job description. She takes them up to Poe Lake on camping trips. Of course, we all know she does it just to chase away weary physicians who might be taking a day's relaxation by fishing."

Wendy, who blushed when anyone talked about her, smiled and gave Doc a loving swat. "Poaching's more like it," she said.

"That's right," Doc said, "every one of those fish in that lake has a patient's name on it and Wendy's job is to make sure no one gets anyone else's personal fish."

Wendy took an instant sisterly fondness for Dr. Rose, and within three days was calling him Rosey.

[3]

Although its name suggested a stylishly decrepit bungalow in a fashionably overgrown setting, Wilson Cottage was hardly even a separate building. It was conceived, built, and named during an era when the plan was to create nearly self-sufficient homelike units within the larger townlike design of the mental hospital. The unit itself was not all that physically different from any other at Bedloe. There were two dormitories, one for men and one for women; two bathrooms; an L-shaped dayroom; and a glass-walled nursing station. Half a dozen staff offices and therapy rooms, plus three seclusion rooms, were distributed along the hallway that linked the unit with the rest of the hospital. Unlike many other wards, Wilson Cottage did have its own door to the parking lot and the hospital grounds.

Wilson Cottage was a so-called open unit, which meant that most of the patients, within certain limits, were free to leave the unit without being accompanied by staff. Most of them, Rosey was somewhat surprised to learn from Wendy, had jobs around the hospital. One woman worked in the hospital beauty shop; two men worked in the carpentry shop, caning chairs and repairing furniture; when their moods allowed it, two women worked as seamstresses, making and repairing clothes; several other men and women worked on the grounds crew, picking up trash and doing housekeeping around the hospital.

Hearing about the jobs, Dr. Rose made the common assumption that this meant that Wilson Cottage's patients were getting progressively better and would someday leave the hospital. Wendy was quick to tell him this was not the case. "One thing you've got to understand," she said. "I have to tell this to all the new staff. They come in here and they're under the impression that these patients in this ward are on their way out of the hospital. You know, like they're real high functioning patients, so any day now they're going to go down and register to vote and never be ill again. This ward isn't like that. Now for some of them, that's true. For most of them, it's not. Most of them don't get better. But they're not bad enough to be put in some of the back wards in the hospital, like D-7 or D-5."

A shiver trembled through Wendy whenever she thought of the D-units.

"I think you're being too pessimistic," Doc said, kindly.

"This is where we fight," Wendy said. "Okay, let me say that a lot of the people here can go either way. But according to the record, they're batting about one hundred. Not exactly all-star material."

Doc nodded, keeping his counsel.

Wendy and Doc introduced Dr. Rose to every patient in Wilson Cottage, but the resident was not good with either names or diagnoses. While some of the patients made distinct and lasting impressions on him, most spun around vaguely in his head: An honest-to-goodness nun who had killed her mother with a crucifix; a young mother who had stabbed, but not killed, her newborn daughter; a former registered nurse at the local medical-surgical hospital who had become psychotic and anesthetized several patients and delivered them for the wrong operations; a schizophrenic man who was in danger of being discharged because his home county was getting tired of paying for his stay at Bedloe; a pleasant-seeming young man who had hitchhiked to the Bedloe Valley from California and killed a man in a bar fight by shoving a beer bottle down his throat; a depressed woman whose husband visited once a month to exercise what he believed were his conjugal rights at a local motel; and a dozen more who remained little more than blurred figures to Steven Rose. He had to refresh his memory by studying their charts whenever he was called upon to work with them.

But there were a few patients at Wilson Cottage Dr. Rose never forgot. One was Greta Lampson, thirty-one years old, a tall, thin, wraith of a woman with long, straight yellow-gray hair, a woman absolutely determined to kill herself. "She's a real tough case, real sad," Wendy said, as she told Rosey about Doc's failed efforts to lift Greta's spirits with antidepressants. "I know Doc wants to try electroshock, but you have to go through an awful lot of legal red tape to be able to do it, since most conservators won't sign the papers."

"A conservator," Wendy explained, "is the person who is responsible for the patient. Since the patients are mentally ill and can't legally make decisions for themselves, they need to have a conservator who can. For most of the people here, the home county is the conservator. That's because their families signed over conservatorship when they couldn't afford to pay the medical and hospital bills. The county takes on the burden, but you have to let them be conservator. That's the way it works. The conservator is supposed to look after the welfare of the patient—and some of them really do that. But most of the time they're trying to save the county's money. It costs something like $100,000 a year to keep a patient in this hospital. So a lot of times the conservators, working for the county, want to get them out of the hospital as soon as possible and get them back to the county facilities where they can take care of them for less money. It's sad. When these people see their conservator coming, they get afraid. They don't want to leave here."

Greta Lampson's conservator, Doc explained, was adamant about refusing permission for electroconvulsive treatments. In this attitude, he was not unique. Most conservators, and many psychiatrists, would rather allow a judge to take the responsibility for ECT, since the judge could not lose his job or be sued if the decision was the wrong one. Greta had two more months on the final antidepressant, then Doc was going to court.

Another sad case that seemed to draw out Steven Rose's sympathy was Mary Johnson, a pretty young black woman with short hair. Mary had lived in a neighborhood where if she walked outside her house the boys would make her take off all her clothes and run around in the street naked. If she refused or resisted, they would beat her. Inside the home she was no safer. Both her father and her uncle regularly raped her. When Rosey gasped at this, Doc pointed out that it was common for young chronic mentally ill people to be sexually abused.

Only twenty-two years old, Mary was a hard case to manage. She spent a lot of time in seclusion, which was a rarity in Wilson Cottage. "She gets into fights a lot," Wendy explained. "Or she just starts yelling at people. She's just scared, that's all. She can be real nice sometimes. I can usually calm her down so she doesn't wind up in the seclusion room." When he first met her, Rosey could not take his eyes off Mary Johnson, who every now and then would slowly wind her head away from the wall and sneak a glance around the room—and then snap it back if she thought someone noticed her.

Rosey asked about Mary Johnson's prognosis. Doc shook his head. Mary had been at Bedloe three months and there had been little progress. "Hard to tell," Doc said. "The tough thing is that even if we get her straightened out somehow, where is she going to go from here? Her best chance is to stay in some kind of institution for the rest of her life. She'd never make it in her old neighborhood. They'll kill her. And if she were discharged from Bedloe, more than likely she'd wind up back home sooner or later. Her county's not real good at funding board and care, which can be a nice sort of halfway house between a hospital and complete discharge."

Then there was Zelda Glover, a short, compact woman in her thirties, with curly black hair and dark eyes that cast suspicion everywhere she looked. Wendy didn't trust Zelda, and Rosey could tell.

"She acts as though she likes me a lot," Wendy explained, "but there's something funny. I don't trust it. She's always wanting to give me presents and do things for me."

"What's wrong with that?" Rosey asked with a frown.

"Nothing. Nothing at all. I guess I don't trust her because I know that some of these people, when they're real crazy, can go from loving you to killing you in a minute."

"You don't have to be crazy to do that. It happens all the time," Rosey said.

"It happens. And it happens," Wendy muttered.

"People are always being killed by their lovers. Heat of passion," Rosey added.

"Funny you should mention that," Wendy said. "That's sort of why Zelda is here. Zelda killed a man she was living with. That's what the judge called it, 'heat of passion.' But they sent her to the hospital because a psychiatrist said she was schizoaffective. I guess that can mean just about anything."

"And does," Doc interjected with a nod and a smile. "Schizoaffective: Schizophrenia with either a rocket engine behind it or a huge stone on top of it. Schizoaffectives don't usually have the social and intellectual disintegration. The delusions and hallucinations are still there, but they can still function, occasionally, if they're not profoundly depressed or manic."

"Sounds like it's hard to tell them apart." Rosey shook his head.

"Damn right it is, sometimes. Lots of people carry both diagnoses in their files," Doc said.

"She spent about two years in the hospital after the murder and then got out," Wendy continued. "Three years later, she got married. Married a wealthy guy. They weren't married more than a year when one day she just jumped on him and stabbed him to death. That was one thing." Wendy paused, as if expecting Rosey to say something like "It happens every day" again. "Then she got scared. There was blood all over the place. She called the emergency police line and . . . when the police arrived Zelda had gotten her needle and thread and was sewing up the body's wounds."

"I see. What's her prognosis?"

"You mean, is she going to get a chance at another husband?" Doc asked with a smile.

Dr. Rose, Doc noticed, seemed impatient with his humor.

"Well, it's anybody's guess," Doc answered. "You always like to be optimistic. The optimistic track for Zelda is that she'll calm down a bit and . . . it's so hard, though. She's got an awful lot of rage in there. Otherwise, she might wind up going after somebody again someday. The thing is that there is an antisocial element in her. No conscience. She can be real cagey. I'd have to say that I'd be equally surprised if she spent the rest of her life in here—or if she were running for governor next election."

Rosey was flustered. "You seem to be describing two ends of the scale! Isn't there a middle road somewhere, a more or less normal, calm, maybe even dull, middle-class life for her that's possible?"

Doc looked at Wendy, who returned his look with raised eyebrows.

"What do you think, Wendy?"

"I guess . . . anything's possible. . . . I just. . . ."

"Wendy's trying to be polite, Rosey. If there's one thing you learn in this business, it's that the middle is pretty much lost to these people. They either somehow find themselves on top if the degree of actual dysfunction is minimal, or, more likely, on the bottom. Our society doesn't allow any middle-class territory for lunatics. They either exalt them or ignore them. But they don't like them living next door. Zelda—or many of the patients in here—could wind up a star, or die a ward of the state. Or maybe both."

"I see," Rosey said. "Tragic. She's a beautiful woman."

The only male patient to hold Dr. Rose's interest was Henry Dove, a gangly fifty-year-old former college professor. He still managed to look professorial, not only because he had a neatly cropped salt-and-pepper beard but also because he was never seen without a book. Henry Dove had actually written two books, scholarly works about European history.

Now all he wanted to do was die. That was his illness. Officially his diagnosis was bipolar disorder, manic-depression. But Doc knew that the essential choice Henry Dove had to make was whether to live or die. Henry wound up at Bedloe after trying to hold up a biker bar with an unloaded gun. "One day he just got so out of control," Wendy explained, "he almost got himself shot, which I guess is what he wanted."

Doc knew Henry had a fair chance at best. Even if he decided he wanted to go back to his life, there would be tremendous obstacles. Doc suspected Henry could make some kind of go at it, but so far he had not been able to help Henry find anything in that life to which he especially wanted to return.

"But he's a sweet, sweet man," Wendy said. "Never a problem."

Dr. Rose, who by midmonth was feeling more a secure part of the Wilson Cottage family—and had even come to like being called Rosey—sat up and shook his head. "I don't understand. Why do you trust Henry when you don't trust Zelda Glover? It seems they both could have carried the same diagnosis if they floated through the system long enough."

"That's right," Doc agreed. "You have a lot of patients who carry diagnoses of schizoaffective and manic-depressive. The boundaries are not always clear. But there is something in the character of their behavior, their history, that just gets you in the guts. Plus, the facts. Zelda has killed two people. Henry went into that bar with a gun that wasn't loaded. He knows the quality of an illusion, knows that an image can be just as dangerous as the real thing. Zelda doesn't know that. Zelda believes her real power is unlimited. Henry knew he had the power to rob the bar and scare people enough to shoot at him—whether or not his gun was loaded. Zelda believed she could sew up her dead husband's wounds and make it all right."

Rosey scratched his head.

"Henry wouldn't hurt anyone," Wendy said, "but himself."

4

Wendy Dixon laid the warm box of muffins on the seat and grabbed the rag to wipe the fog off the inside of the windshield. It was one of those damp mornings when the defroster on the old Ford pickup would only make it worse until the engine heated up. By then she would be down the mountain, on the grounds of the hospital and as good as parked in her usual space behind Wilson Cottage. Of course, Wendy reminded herself, she was actually on the grounds of the hospital right now. Bedloe owned the land across the street from her house and all the way down the mountain, for the entire ten-minute drive.

Wendy reminded herself to remember to put one of the muffins aside to eat that night in the middle of the loneliest part of her second double shift in a week.

She stiffened when she saw a snowy stretch of road up ahead. There was always more snow up here than down below, even though there wasn't much more than a thousand-foot difference in altitude. It was time to slow down again anyway. Poe Lake was coming up.

Every morning on her way to work—actually, whenever she drove by—Wendy slowed or stopped by Poe Lake and took a good look around for trespassers. The lake was on the hospital grounds and had been developed as a recreational area for the patients. In its heyday it had been the scene of grand parties and barbecues. There was a cabin large enough to contain a kitchen and dining room, a cozy parlor with a huge fireplace constructed of local stones, and a dance floor. The cabin was ringed by a wide, screened porch. Nearer the lake there was a wooden pavilion and picnic area at least as big as the cabin. The five-acre lake had originally been stocked and the bank nearest the road landscaped to allow fishing. A small pier and boat launch were the final touches.

The entire complex was now in disrepair. All the buildings were still strong and safe, thanks to the way they built things half a century ago. But there were a lot of little things that needed to be done: walls painted, small leaks patched, torn screens and broken windows replaced, lights and plumbing repaired, overgrown grass and shrubbery trimmed. The present hospital administration did nothing to maintain the grounds. Whenever Wendy or the staff of another unit wanted to bring a party of patients to the lake, they not only had to get special permission, but they also had to pay the hospital grounds crew out of their own pockets to cut the jungle down to manageable size.

But the property belonged to the patients—it had been built for them, and some of them still used it. That's why Wendy always slowed down and focused her sharp eyes on the banks of the lake. As much as the place had been neglected, Mother Nature had seen to it that the lake remained well-stocked. Almost no townspeople knew that fact, and only a few of the hospital staff. But every now and then Wendy would spot a few people fishing or having a party. Then she would go into action and chase them off. Nicely, of course. First she would explain that this area belonged to the patients and was for their use. That usually worked on hospital staff. Now and then a stubborn doctor all decked out in full fishing gear would have to be asked his name for reporting to the hospital police—but that was rare. The hospital police had enough trouble keeping wandering patients inside the grounds without having to worry about a few trespassers. Luckily, the doctor never seemed to want his name to appear on a list that would come to the attention of the administration.

Townspeople were the most difficult to chase off. When polite words didn't work, and they knew the hospital police weren't worth a spit in the wind, Wendy could usually dislodge them by telling them that if they weren't going to leave, could they please just try not to disturb the large party of patients that was going to be coming up any minute now.

Wendy slowed the truck and peered down the short dirt driveway to the lake. There were no tracks in the snow, and Wendy saw nothing moving around the cabin or the lake.

She stopped the truck. Something had moved on the ground among the bare trees near the path between the lake and the cabin.

Without taking her eyes off the spot, Wendy shut off the engine and got out of the truck. The woods were quieter than they should have been.

She crossed the street and started down the dirt road, scanning for more signs of movement.

There it was again. This time she saw what it was: a crow hopping around. Maybe it was wounded.

No, there were two crows there and something on the ground.

Obviously, nobody was fishing or disturbing anything on the grounds. Whatever was going on was apparently well within the bounds of nature taking its course. A wounded bird or a dead animal in the snow. But Wendy was curious. Maybe a poacher had left his catch behind?

She was close enough now to see that it was bigger than a fish or two. Maybe a wounded deer shot on the other side of the mountain had come here to die.

Wendy stopped short, and turned away to look for a tree to lean against. It was a person she saw there, a human body. She looked again, and it was what she thought it was.

The woods were so quiet now that the sound of the black wings' fluttering was loud enough to frighten Wendy. She was confused. She felt like running, but she had to chase those damn birds away. A person's body couldn't be carrion. Besides, chasing the crows away gave her an excuse to scream. She ran at them, waving her arms and screaming, trying not to let her eyes focus on the body.

But when the crows were gone, Wendy was right there, just off the path, and the body, a woman's, was right in front of her, dressed only in a tattered slip of snow. Her skin had taken on a sickly bluish tint and there were green-black bruises here and there. Wendy couldn't take her eyes off her. The woman's last conscious act as a living creature had been to try to cover her eyes with her hands, and now, in death, her fingers had stiffened and clawed over her open eyes. Wendy recognized her, from her wispy blond hair, mostly. She was a patient in one of the "back" wards, D-5, known to be one of the worst in the hospital. Wendy had filled in there a few times. When she had given the patients their medications, the young woman with the wispy blond hair had twice as many pills as any of the others. Yet she had smiled when Wendy gave her the pills. Had she been the one who kept moaning all night about her lost little baby?

The sobs started to come, shaking Wendy from the inside. The problem was, she had to get help but she didn't want to leave the poor girl here all alone. The crows had just flown to a nearby tree and were patiently waiting for Wendy to leave.

5 _____

[1]

We are not rational, orderly creatures by nature. Our sails fill with the winds of emotion and carry our flimsy crafts across seas of desire and fear. Reason is a little rudder, but where the primeval forces that shape and quicken the psyche utter only guttural moans and sighs as they are about their work, reason has the use of language. Reason loves words, and will fling them in the face of whatever storms and earthquake tides threaten from above and below. We need reason to navigate, we need the things it begets with its love of words, things like rules, bylaws, regulations, and data. Fortunately, language has other children, so we also get poetry and song.

The National Medical Accreditation Committee, which had inspected Bedloe State Hospital two years earlier, had no use for poetry or song. Faced with a human enterprise as storm-tossed as the state mental hospital, the committee mustered an army of words and marched them into neat columns for the attack on chaos. How

else to examine such a confused business as the care of profoundly
ill people?

Of course, the committee was interested in the actual physical
details of care. Its members were concerned that patients were as
comfortable, clean, and well cared for as modern medical science
allowed. But they were first interested in how these details were
represented in words. So the committee did not immediately look
for dirty hallways or neglected patients. They marched their columns of words through the hospital records looking for the Enemy.
They assumed that whenever words were missing from expected
places, such as patient records, the Enemy had won a victory.

Only after every available record was inspected did the committee officially raise its eyes from the paper and look around at the
hospital. Perhaps they did this last because they knew appearances
were the easiest to fake. Even the most slovenly administrator, if he
was clever, could perform cosmetic miracles. Most administrators
were neither altogether slovenly nor consummately clever. Sam
Akbar, superintendent of Bedloe State Hospital, was not distinguished in either category.

The National Medical Accreditation Committee was not without
controversy itself. It had been criticized and attacked by both
medical-consumer groups and hospital organizations. Consumer
groups said it was too lenient in its evaluations, that it failed to
decertify hospitals that performed poorly, and that by keeping its
evaluations from the public eye it allowed dangerous situations to
persist. Hospital organizations charged that the committee inspectors exaggerated trivial problems.

Nevertheless, the committee continued to be the single most
powerful medical certification body in the country. Its word controlled billions of dollars in private, state, and federal money for
health care—not only for state hospitals like Bedloe, but also for
private mental hospitals, as well as for municipal and private
medical-surgical hospitals. Without accreditation, a hospital could
be cut off from huge chunks of its operating budget. Several private
hospitals and even a few state and municipal hospitals were known
to have closed within weeks of decertification by the committee.

Bedloe State Hospital had not fared well in its most recent
inspection by the committee, two years earlier. Administrative records were in cleverly arranged shambles. The inspectors privately

commented that Bedloe seemed to have the organizational structure of a clumsy Third-World dictatorship. The condition of the medical staff, however, made the hospital's organizational structure look efficient by comparison.

The committee was concerned that the physicians be organized into a "staff" which met regularly, made rules and regulations governing professional work, reviewed performance, and kept adequate records of what was going on in the hospital and with its patients. It was understandable that the committee should want the values of the physician to dominate, since the committee had been founded by physicians and was still composed mostly of physicians. That physicians be at least a nominally self-governing body inside the hospital was a traditional standard that had been established three-quarters of a century earlier, during a time when the physician's absolute authority in medical affairs was hardly ever questioned.

For more than a quarter century, Bedloe's psychiatrists had not been organized into a "medical staff" at all. They had less professional organization than a crew of cowboys, who at least could share information, express grievances, and plan rebellion in the bunkhouse. The committee found Bedloe's doctors to be a confused, alienated bunch of medical day laborers.

That was why the position of medical director had been created and Alex Greco hired to fill it.

Bedloe had not been exactly decertified, but had been put on probation. This was a frequent tactic of the committee. It usually allowed a hospital to stay open as long as it was making progress toward full certification. The committee's critics charged that this allowed marginal and sometimes dangerous institutions to remain open. The committee, however, was acting within a centuries-old tradition that dictated a "collegial" approach when pointing out deficiencies to a fellow physician.

[2]

Alex Greco held in his mind a single image of his boss, Sam Akbar. It wasn't his first, but it was the one that came alive in his imagination whenever he thought about Sam. A couple of days after Akbar had hired him, they went on a tour of the hospital. Alex made

careful note of the way staff grew suspiciously mechanical around
the slim, wiry man with fine, straight, gray-brown hair and bird-like
facial features. After the tour, back in Alex's office, Akbar sat down in
Alex's chair behind the desk, shook his head and grimaced. He
screwed his head around to look directly at Alex, who was standing
on the other side of his desk, and nodded.

"I've worked with retards," Sam said. "And I've worked with
crazies. And I'll take retards every time."

Sam Akbar had survived his way up through the ranks from
supply clerk to become superintendent of a relatively small state
hospital for penal-code patients across the state from Bedloe County. When he learned of the vacancy at Bedloe, he had managed to be
on the phone with the state director of mental health about matters
having nothing to do with the hospital. Still, they wound up talking
about Bedloe, and Akbar was named the new boss two weeks later.

Bedloe, already severely troubled long before Akbar took over,
got worse under his leadership. In its report, the committee cited
the fact that there was no medical authority at all in the hospital.
Physicians reported to nonmedical supervisors and, ultimately, to
the superintendent, who had no medical training at all. The committee's impending decision on accreditation, which would be
rendered after its next inspection, scheduled for September, meant
tens of millions of dollars to the hospital. Medicare and dozens of
other third-party payers would not pay for care at the hospital if it
lost its accreditation. Alex Greco had been hired to mollify the
committee.

Citing its requirement that certain aspects of hospital care had to
be overseen by a physician, the committee had demanded that the
hospital create the position of medical director in order to give
physicians a permanent role in the administration and to bring the
medical aspects of patient care up to acceptable medical standards.
The administration's plan was to hire a psychiatrist and put him in
nominal charge of the physicians.

From the first, Alex sensed that Sam Akbar's idea was to isolate
him from any real authority in the hospital at large and thus limit his
power to make real changes. So he had purposely not rattled cages
too much during his first year at Bedloe. He had, instead, gained a
picture of the way things worked—and it wasn't a pretty sight. He
had found the administration's style to be one of bureaucratic bul-

lying and manipulation. The bullying had taken its toll on the psychiatrists: Alex found them a ragtag, disheveled bunch whose morale was so low that they were deficient in carrying out even the responsibilities which were theirs by law, not to mention those demanded by their professional oath.

During his first year Alex had been inundated day and night by psychiatrists seeking his approval for routine psychiatric treatment matters. His home was no refuge: the phone rang at least twice every evening, and often in the middle of the night. On these occasions Alex would listen to the psychiatrist on the other end talk about some crisis that had come up. Usually a patient was seriously decompensating, which meant whatever stabilization had been reached, usually through medication, was now failing and the patient's thinking and behavior were becoming perilously disorganized.

Alex would listen carefully and get as much information as he could. He would try to draw out the psychiatrist and lead him as far as possible from the language of a bureaucrat shuffling responsibility toward that of a seasoned physician. And then, finally, when all the information was revealed and both physicians had discussed alternatives and the course of action had become apparent, Alex would say, "You're the doctor."

There was usually a moment in which the psychiatrist on the other end of the line would mutter an almost silent statement of amazement . . . and then Alex would repeat, "You're the doctor." And that would be the end of it.

As Alex's medical staff learned to take the responsibility they were trained for, morale was resurrected and the nighttime calls gradually diminished, until now the only calls he received were genuine emergencies too hot to be handled without the medical director's immediate attention, and even these occurred only about twice a week. In less than a year, Alex had accomplished one of his primary goals: he had restored professional pride to the almost one hundred psychiatrists under him, men and women who had had it beaten out of them by a system that depended on physicians, but did everything in its power to demean them.

Naturally, there were bad apples, too, physicians who plainly did not belong in a mental hospital. These doctors were easy to spot. You could look at their patients' charts and see the signs of poor care or outright neglect. You could observe the way the staff acted around them. Staff usually had good things to say about, and around, a good physician. With a poor one they were more cautious and rarely made eye contact when talking to him or about him.

Alex didn't like to fire doctors. Usually, putting them on notice that they were being watched was enough. They got the hint that Bedloe was no longer a good place to hide and found other jobs. You needed a damn good issue to fire a doctor. The trouble you got afterward could be immense.

There was plenty more to be done to bring Bedloe up to medical standards, but even the little Alex had already done had drawn Akbar's suspicion, so Alex knew he was being watched very closely.

Nevertheless, this was the year Alex was planning to emerge from his relative slumber and start to make some real changes. This was the year the committee would be coming back to Bedloe. Alex knew that as far as Sam was concerned, enough had already been done to satisfy the committee's specific demands. But he also knew that Akbar was probably wrong.

Alex had no crusade in mind, but was just going about his business as a physician. His ambition was to serve well. But whatever his employers may have believed, he was always aware of a higher allegiance, a set of standards older and more deeply rooted than those of the state. The state really didn't care about medical ethics as long as the business of the state was moving along. The state had its own standards and only as much compassion as had been legislated and supported in the budget. Sam was a creature of such standards, but Alex was not. And as soon as Akbar had discovered this about Alex, the two men became opponents in an undeclared war, one which Alex feared would inevitably reach a climax when Akbar would ask for his resignation.

But it was not to be just yet, that Alex knew. The discovery of the female patient's body at Poe Lake would draw enough attention to the hospital. The dismissal or resignation of a member of the administration at the same time would increase attention to an unmanageable degree. Alex would not even have to make any accusations or fight his dismissal. All he would have to do would be to hire an attorney and hold a press conference. That would be enough to raise the media clamor to a fever pitch and would most likely result in some kind of state investigation of the hospital. Alex and Sam and everyone else involved in state institutions had seen it happen several times. Nobody in the current administration of the hospital ever benefited from such feeding frenzies. There was already enough blood in the water, and Sam couldn't chance some of his own catching the sensitive noses of the predators out there.

Alex knew from experience that Sam Akbar preferred not to investigate violent incidents too closely. Akbar had not survived twenty-three years in the state department of mental health by investigating things closely.

Alex didn't need an investigation. He knew what the problem was: Dean Lester, M.D., the physician responsible for units D-7, the male long-term chronic ward, and D-5, the female long-term chronic ward where the murdered patient had lived. Alex knew that Lester was so deficient at practicing medicine and psychiatry that in the past year three of his patients had died from purely medical problems and six from suicide.

Lester's units were the pits of the hospital, and they needed to be cleaned up badly. And they could be, too, Alex knew.

But it wasn't going to happen any time soon. Alex had pressed for some changes, but Akbar said the patient's murder would not provoke much of an investigation, and he could handle it. That meant he could prevent the investigation from penetrating the hospital and exposing the true state of units D-7 and D-5. "Now that you've done such a good job and raised morale among the physicians," Akbar had said, "there really is no need to tempt fate and go any further."

Alex knew Akbar was wrong—but he also knew that in the weeks before the committee's next visit, in September, Sam would send in the carpenters to repair the broken and decrepit furniture and walls and windows and give the hospital a coat of new paint. The patients would all receive new clothes and the treatment teams would go over every patient's record so the chart would have some new sheets of paper in it. And when the investigators came, the place would be bright and sparkling and the patients cleaned up.

And Bedloe would pass. Maybe.

Alex shook his head to dispel the poison. His eyes were drawn to one of the paintings on his wall, one of a seventeenth-century European mental hospital. The picture depicted a women's ward. It was a warm summer day and the patients were in the courtyard sitting on benches or on the ground. At first glance most of the women appeared well-dressed in the fashion of the day, which included billowing skirts and blouses. But looking again, more closely, you saw the rags, saw the women clutching at their clothing, tearing it off, exposing their breasts. Looking more closely still you saw their faces, eyes downcast in misery and shame, or on fire with anguished wantonness. A tall, stately physician walks in the yard, and some of the women watch him. Some are too ill to escape their hallucinations, some too miserable to open their eyes to the light of day. All of the women, the fat and skinny, the beautiful despite their madness, are chained. One of them has crawled over to the physician and is embracing his ankle and about to kiss his leg.

What had always fascinated Alex about his own painting was that the physician is obviously moved, but not overwhelmed. He has compassion for these wretched human beings, but he also has the strength to help them—and he will help them. Their curse is not his curse; it does not mean to him that the race is cursed. This man has faith.

Alex had such faith at one time, and this painting could remind him of it. Today, all it did was prompt him to leave his office and start the drive home a little early, and, perhaps, keep something of himself in reserve for the fight he knew would come, must come, if he was to continue to call himself a physician.

[3]

The foot or more of February snow absorbed all background sounds and gave the hospital the still air of a graveyard. But Alex knew the stones harbored life that watched and listened and waited, so he was always a little tense walking from his office to his car. The tension did not ease until he was in the Lincoln and rolling down the tree-lined avenue from the administration building to the front gate. Then he could take a deep, free, easy breath at last.

So there would be no real investigation of the death of the woman whose body was found at Poe Lake. Woman? She was somewhere between fifteen and twenty-two and barely had the chance to fight the normal battles of girlhood. She called herself Deborah Smith. Not quite a year ago she had gotten off an interstate bus in one of the far counties of the state and gone stone catatonic right on the spot. She had no money, no luggage, and no identification. Deborah Smith was brought to Bedloe, where Alex began an investigation. The police in the bus's originating city in another state had no record of a missing person answering to her description. The local mental health center first said they had no information, then said they had no information they could give out. After Alex pressed them, they admitted that the laws of confidentiality prohibited them from giving out any information about any of their patients.

Deborah Smith was a treatment by bus ticket. As Alex cruised over the mountain and felt the Lincoln escape gravity for an instant as it came over the crest and left the Bedloe Valley behind, he constructed her history: He could tell she had not been raised in poverty. She had been well-nourished and kept clean. Her teeth were white and healthy. There were no signs of a sordid childhood. Deborah was most likely the child of solidly middle-class parents. She probably had her first breakdowns in her teens. In the midst of the normal adolescent storms, the hundred-year hurricane broke inside her mind and tore her life apart. And the life of her parents, who had not the slightest idea what to do.

At some point she had run away, wound up bouncing from one community mental health center to another. Maybe she went home during one of her calmer periods. Probably not. This one was so young and so ill that she probably went off the scale within the first year or two. The community mental health centers would not be able to handle her. Many of them had psychiatrists on part-time duty at best. Finally, a center whose resources were already pushed to the limit simply stripped her of identification—if she even had any by that point—and put her on a bus. It was done every day. Bedloe not only received such castoffs, but it also contributed its share back to the flow.

After a week on medication at Bedloe, the girl said, "My name was Deborah Smith," already referring to herself in the past tense.

"Her name was Deborah Smith," Alex said out loud as he made the turn for his street.

Alex didn't want Deborah Smith's life to end that way. He thought of her parents' agony, never knowing what happened to their little girl. Their mystery was so much more immense than the mechanical details of her death. Alex felt a physical hunger for an investigation. He wanted it to be like a mystery novel, wanted there to be heroes and villains, and a murderer who could stand in for the focus of evil in this drama. He wanted something to intrude on the common reality and give it a meaning that was in some way more: more horrible, more political, more glamorous, more frightening, more mysterious, more satisfying.

Alex knew there was no mystery.

At Bedloe State Hospital there were more than one hundred assaults per week. Patients assaulting patients. Patients assaulting staff. Staff assaulting patients. Most were minor scuffles, tempers worn thin by illness or stress, or incidents where staff got a bit too rough in subduing a patient. Many were more or less accidents.

But then there were the outright attacks that seemed to come from nowhere. A physician, psych tech, social worker, or psychologist would walk into a ward and a patient would simply attack. Sometimes more patients would join in, on one side or the other. And there were killings, an average of two per year, not counting the twenty or thirty "medical deaths" and two or three dozen suicides.

It was very plain what had happened: This helpless child was not taken care of and had become a victim of natural forces. Concentrating on the minute details of the last two or three acts that chased life from her body was just a ploy to ignore the general complicity. Deborah Smith was not killed by a focus of evil, but by a blandness of responsibility. She was a sacrifice.

Alex was home, trudging through snow that held open the gate of the white picket fence, and the phone was ringing.

6

[1]

Fran Channing fought to will the hesitation out of her steps down the corridors of Bedloe State Hospital. She knew from experience that in mental hospitals, doors that were supposed to be locked were not always locked.

Back home at the county L facility where, two years ago, Walter had languished for several months, there was always an open door, even if the L stood for locked. Fran always smiled bitterly at the way people called a locked facility an L facility—as if the L didn't mean what it meant, but, instead, meant that it was just one of many different kinds of facilities, some of which were N facilities, some M facilities, and some L. But there were no N or M facilities, or O or P or Q facilities either—only L's.

Fran paused and looked around for a sign. The Receiving Unit where Walter had spent his first weeks was in a wing of this building. That ward had surprised Fran. It was cleaner, brighter, and more efficient than Fran had expected. The psych tech who welcomed Walter seemed both kind and able. She had taken Fran and Brad aside and told them that it would not be unusual for their son to get sicker for a week or two immediately after the move, but that he would be closely watched and well cared for until he settled down and adjusted to the hospital routines. Then he would be moved to his permanent home in the hospital.

Fran had heard similar well-meaning lectures, but she still bristled at the sound of the words "permanent home," even though she knew the tech meant "permanent" only in relation to Walter's "temporary" stay in the Receiving Unit. Walter had only one real home.

As predicted, Walter had gotten sicker that first week, Fran learned through telephone calls to the unit. But he settled down and was moved to his home unit after three weeks.

This was Fran's first visit since Walter's admission. She had wanted to come earlier but a series of late winter storms kept the roads treacherous. When she finally called to ask about coming in, the woman who answered the phone on the ward had told her the physician would have to approve her visit and that he would call her back. Fran waited three days, then called again. She was assured the psychiatrist would call at his earliest opportunity. She asked how Walter was doing, but the woman on the other end shouted at someone in the room and hung up the phone. Fran called back. This time there was no answer. She waited a day before calling again. This time a different person answered, someone named Randy, who told Fran to come in the following week. Randy told her that she was just a fill-in on the unit, that she didn't know the patients very well, but that she would tell the doctor Fran was coming in.

There were no signs. Fran decided she might as well try to ask someone. She picked a short, matronly woman with gray-blue hair, who was carrying some papers down the hall.

"Excuse me, can you tell me how to find unit D-7?"

The woman stopped and looked at Fran. For a brief instant she was afraid the woman was going to tell her to leave, but then she smiled and gave her directions. Fran followed them and soon found herself looking down a long hall and knowing Walter was somewhere at the end of it. The floor was so polished Fran could see her distorted reflection in it, so that she was a ghost moving across a narrow, nightmare dance floor. The walls were completely barren: no doors, no windows, no decorations. Rather, they were a dull tan from which the enthusiasm of color had been stolen.

The doors at the end were brown, and beyond them, a darkness. These doors should be locked, Fran knew, but they looked ajar. She opened the door quickly.

There was another hallway, this one short and dark. On her left she passed a closed door with the word Storage painted on it in square letters. She could hear voices now, and water running behind the door ahead and to her right. Fran caught sight of movement ahead in the gloom, where the hall seemed to open up into a larger space. The sound of running water grew suddenly louder as the door to her right swung open. A man came through the open door with his pants down. When he saw Fran he stopped and stared at her. Fran saw beyond him into the bathroom, where a thin layer of gray water crept over the tile floor.

In the bathroom a man screamed. Fran turned away and continued down the hall. Directly in front of her was a small room with glass walls, the nursing station. The room was a dim island of light in the murky gray up ahead, so Fran focused on it as she advanced. There were some people in the room, and one of them, a middle-aged woman, was looking at Fran while taking a quick, intense drag on a cigarette, exhaling, and filling the room with her smoke.

"The door was left unlocked again, people," the woman said, still looking at Fran, spitting out wisps of smoke with every word.

The other people in the nursing station, a tall, thin man dressed in athletic warmups and a younger woman who was also smoking, now came to the glass to look at Fran. Fran kept going.

When she was close to the nursing station she could see beyond it, and what she saw stopped her. The hall opened up into a much larger room, a dismal beehive. Despite the dark—no lights were on and little came through the windows—the tumult in the room forced Fran back like a blast from a volcano. Dozens of men half-dressed in pajamas tops or bottoms, men undressed, men sloppily dressed in torn, filthy clothing paced back and forth in front of her. One of them seemed to be silently explaining something to an imaginary person. As he paced, he whispered and gesticulated over and over with great energy and emphasis. Another man kept jabbing the air in front of his face. Another clapped his hands.

There was no organized structure to the macabre dance. Every man had chosen a direction different from all the others, if even by a couple of degrees, and was mechanically following it as if he were on a rail. Nobody bumped into anybody else.

"Can I help you, Ma'am?" The middle-aged woman from the nursing station had come out and was grimacing disapprovingly at Fran.

Fran tried to look at her, but her attention was riveted to the room, searching for Walter. There were couches along the wall and dozens more men slouched on them like rag dolls. Some were dressed, some not. Several of them had their hands casually extended down the front or back of their pants.

The man in the bathroom screamed again. Several of the men looked over, and a few seemed to become more agitated. "Uh oh, uh oh, uh oh," murmured one.

"Billy, check that out, will ya?" the woman in front of Fran shouted back at the others.

"Sure, Penny." The younger woman took a last slow drag on her cigarette and crushed it in an ashtray as she got up from her chair and swaggered lazily out of the nursing station.

"Can I help you, Ma'am?" the middle-aged woman said to Fran again. She had gray-blond overcurled hair that didn't seem natural for her head. Her eyes inspected Fran disapprovingly.

"I'm here to see my son, Walter Channing."

"That's not possible, Ma'am. This is a locked unit. You'll have to leave." As she spoke, the woman moved her stocky body in front of Fran, blocking her view.

Fran noticed that none of the men had shoes on. Several of them had stopped pacing now and were staring at her. One man's face twitched uncontrollably. A short, fat man sat down and started to sob. The man in the bathroom screamed again.

Fran looked at the woman's eyes, which were widening expectantly. The woman tucked her chin down and put her hand on her hip, which was cocked to one side. Then Fran surprised herself. Later, she would wonder why she said it, why the psych tech's hostility managed to push her to a level of primitive response that she would never have expected existed in herself. It was also true that Fran would come to rely on it more and more, to hold her position or win precious inches of new ground in the war of attrition her life had become. Fran was suddenly stripped of all reason and diplomacy, and could say only one thing:

"I'm not leaving until I see my son."

The woman, Penny, shifted her weight to the other hip, and switched hands, too. She kept her eyes on Fran, who did not move.

A man in gray, dirty unbuttoned pajamas shuffled up. "I'm hungry, Penny. I ain't had no breakfast. I ain't had no breakfast today."

Penny ignored him. Both women's eyes were locked on each other. "Well," Penny started, "I'm gonna hafta call security."

"What seems to be the problem here?" A tall, portly man draped in a tentlike white coat towered over Fran and the psych tech. Fran could hear his labored, raspy breath as if he were drawing from and expelling air right into her ear. His eyes were blue slits in his pink face, and they seemed to smile kindly on Fran.

"I'm Fran Channing. I'm here to see my son, Walter Channing. I called last week."

"Oh, yes! Of course." As he spoke, he put his hand on the psych tech's shoulder. "Randy told me you were coming in."

"Nobody told me about this. Nobody told me," Penny spat as she shook her head.

"I'll take care of Mrs. Channing, Penny," the fat man said.

Penny swaggered away, her head down and shaking. "I wish people would tell me about these things. I'm only the supervisor around here." She went back into the nursing station and flopped down into a chair, still shaking her head.

"Mrs. Channing, I am Dr. Dean Lester, at your service. I'm your son's psychiatrist here." He extended his hand. Fran took it and weakly gave it a perfunctory shake.

"My son, Walter, was moved here from the Receiving Unit last month and I wanted to see him and—"

"Of course you do. That's perfectly all right. Do you see him . . . here, I mean?"

Fran had not seen Walter. But she could only steal glances around the room while confronted by Penny Scott. Now, with the psychiatrist's permission, she scanned the room again, slowly.

The scene was a panorama of misery and chaos. There must have been between forty and fifty men in the room and not a single eye in the room was making contact with any other. Men stared at the ceiling, at the floor, at their own clothes, at nothing. Men slumped on the sofas along the wall had their eyes closed and their mouths open. Several sitting on the floor shifted their eyes nervously around the room. Because she could not pull her eyes away from them, Fran looked at every face longer than she had to in order to see if it was Walter or not.

Is this what her son was, Fran thought to herself as her horror mounted? Is this what he would always be? She knew the answer was more than yes, because there was something of Walter in each of these men. Each one of them had a mother, too, and suddenly Fran felt she might swoon, for she could sense all the pain as if she were the mother of them all.

The sensation passed. On closer inspection, Fran saw that what she had thought was one large room was actually two rooms. The room to the right was separated from this one by a wall that was glass from about three feet high upward. There were so many men pacing and walking and milling about both rooms that, in the gloom, Fran had not seen the wall or the wide doorway into it.

She glanced at the doctor and took a few tentative steps. "I don't see him in this room, Doctor."

He followed her without a word, so Fran kept going. The patient who had complained of hunger—and who had not moved—also followed. "Are we going to eat now? I ain't had no breakfast. I ain't had no breakfast."

Fran walked slowly, so she could track her progress and not collide with any of the pacing men. She stopped to let one pass, a short, thin, intense young man with black hair who was staring at his hands, which he held out in front of his face and nervously spindled as he walked. He stopped right in front of her. Through his wildly spindling fingers he asked Fran, "Who are you? Hmmmmmm? Hmmmmmm? Hmmmmmm?"

"I'm Walter's mother."

"My mother is Marilyn Monroe. No, my mother is Penny Scott. My mother is Penny Scott!" The man's eyes narrowed and sparkled mischievously. He said it louder, "My mother is Penny Scott!" That brought an explosion of sarcastic laughter from the nursing station. Pleased, the man continued pacing.

There were only three men on the couch in the other dayroom. A television was on, but was ignored. One man was sleeping face down on the floor, Fran could tell from his straight, shaggy black hair and paunchy body that he was not Walter. The other men were holding their heads in their hands and rocking back and forth.

Fran was suddenly glad that her husband, Brad, had not come. She knew this would be too much for him. He had gone with her the day the county car brought Walter to Bedloe. They drove up behind it all the way to the hospital. Brad went in with her to the Receiving Unit. That was the same as this—but it was so different. It was the same because, now she remembered, it was laid out the same, with a large dayroom and a nursing station. Patients paced and gesticulated and sobbed and sat on the floor there, too. Some were even in restraints. But most of them were dressed, and those who were not had a full set of pajamas on. And there was light in that ward.

No shades were drawn over the windows, and yet the light seemed not to want to come into this place. All Fran could see were gray bushes and shadows when she looked out the windows.

Fran turned to leave the room, and remembered Dr. Lester. "My son is not in here."

Lester gently took her arm and led her through the room to the door on the other side, "He must still be in bed," he said, as if they had been stupid to suspect otherwise.

The door led into a dormitory, a long, dull room with single beds thrust out from the wall, barracks style, spaced only far enough apart to squeeze in tall gray lockers. Fran was immediately struck by the odor of urine. The beds were unmade, sheets and blankets were clumped and draped every which way across the beds and on the floor. She heard a click behind her and a burst of light from the overhead fluorescent bulbs flashed and died, flashed again, and finally caught, filling the room with a sickly half-light. Not all the bulbs lit. Several buzzed and continued to flicker. One burned a dull red.

Fran searched each bed, each individual island of disarray, each clump of sheet and blanket, for her son, counting the beds from one to the next. As if he had read her mind, Lester interrupted her concentration, "There are thirty-five beds in this dorm and twenty-five in the other."

Fran turned to him. "You have sixty patients in this ward?"

"Yes. Right now we're at full capacity."

Fran resumed her search by walking down the aisle between the ends of the beds. Some of the clumps were so bulky they could easily have hidden a man. None did.

There was no door at the end of the row. Anticipating her again, Lester reached for Fran's arm and ushered her back toward the other side of the room. "The other dorm is across the dayroom. You see, these were originally set up to be two semiseparate units, with one nursing station between them."

Walking back through the beehive, Fran scanned for a gloomy corner she might have missed. She checked every shadowy face once again. This time she felt more of the eyes in the room were following her.

"You hurt Tom! You hurt Tom!" cried a middle-aged man with a salt-and-pepper stubble on his chin. Fran stopped, thinking he was talking to her. But he ignored her as he shuffled indignantly away from a younger man who was slouched on the sofa.

"Is it always so dark in here, Doctor?" Fran finally asked.

"Well, several of the patients are on medications that render their eyes photosensitive. That means the light hurts their eyes."

"Doc, when we gonna eat?" a short, curly-haired man whose eyes appeared clearer and more alert than the rest said as he waved at Lester.

"Be patient, Robby," Lester replied in a fatherly way.

Fran wanted to ask him if the patients had eaten breakfast yet, but she didn't want to press too hard at this point. She was counting on the psychiatrist's cooperation to find her son. Although she knew she had a perfect right to be there, since she had an appointment, and that it was the physician's responsibility to know where her son was, the atmosphere of the ward had weakened her, clipped some of her self-respect and drained her expectations, until all she could focus on right now was finding Walter.

The other dormitory was a duplicate of the first, only a little larger. The same two messy rows of unmade beds, and the same acrid smell of bed linen wet with urine greeted Fran at the door. She searched the tangled mounds, hesitating as long as she could before setting out down the aisle. And then she saw the feet sticking out from a bed about two-thirds down the row.

"Walter?" she whispered. She took a deep breath. "Walter?" she said with more volume.

Fran started for the bed. "Walter!" she cried, almost shouting, already inspecting what she could see of the form on the bed, watching for familiar signs, the funny shape of his big toe, the scar on his right calf where he fell off his bicycle when he was ten.

The scar was not there.

"This isn't my son," Fran exhaled as if it were her last breath. She was about to sit down on the nearest bed, but the odor of urine stopped her.

"Let's go back to the nursing station, Mrs. Channing. Perhaps he was sent out for some . . . some kind of routine . . . test or . . ." Lester didn't finish his sentence, and he started walking away from Fran without his previous courtesies of ushering her out.

Back in the dayroom, the cramped, claustrophobic buzz intensified as if in response to Lester's embarrassed urgency. As he took long, hurried strides through the room, the men seemed to part for him. The pacers stopped short and took a step or two back. The men who had been sitting on the floor leaned and crawled out of his way, including one who was smearing feces in his hair.

And the people in the nursing station quickened to his approach. He hurried in and spoke rapidly in a low voice to Penny. As she listened, Penny's eyes focused dully on Fran, who was just emerging from the dormitory. Fran saw the woman's eyes sharpen on her for just an instant before they became aware that Fran saw them—then they dulled again.

Fran felt all the eyes on her now. Even Lester's, whose lips seemed to move faster the closer Fran got to the nursing station. Penny strode out of the nursing station and turned down the hall. Lester came out to meet Fran.

"Apparently your son was sent out for some tests. Penny is going to check to see if he's ready to come back. This happens all the time. . . ."

Fran was listening to what he said, but she was drawn into Penny's wake. If that woman was going to where Walter was, she was going to follow her.

Lester caught up with her after a few steps down the hall, right in front of the bathroom door, and put his hand on her shoulder, gently, but firmly enough to stop her.

"Penny will be back in a moment. Why don't you come back to the nurses' station, Mrs. Channing."

Fran said nothing. A wide, shiny damp spot mushroomed out from the bathroom door where the floor had been mopped. The sickeningly sweet smell of disinfectant hit Fran in waves. When each wave receded, the stench of the toilet overflow came back. Fran's head began to spin. She tightened her fingers into two fists and stood solidly. The doctor was about to sweep her away, but she felt that if his arm came around her she might relax back into his grip and swoon. She shrugged his arm off her.

"Dr. Lester, I don't understand how you could lose my son like this!"

Lester didn't answer right away. In that silence, watching his face and waiting, Fran understood that they really had lost Walter. They really did not know where her son was. The psych tech had been sent on a fishing expedition, but they had not even a clue where he really was.

Fran was silent with the recognition. Then she gave over her self-control to her mother's instincts. She took several deep breaths, the last one the deepest, and wailed as loud as she could, filling her cry with all her mother's pain and alarm and anguish, "WAAALLL-TERRRR!"

For a moment there was a hush in the beehive, then a scattering of grunts and groans. "Waaalllterrrr!" one man wailed back. "Walter! Walter! Walter!" another one shouted. The buzz came back louder, and cries of "Walter!" punctuated it.

Fran felt she might burst, or faint, or just cry.

"Maaamaaa!"

Fran heard it, and Lester heard it, too.

"Maaama!"

It wasn't coming from the beehive.

"Maaama!"

It was coming from the bathroom.

Fran was through the doorway in an instant. "Walter! I'm coming!" The room was cold and there were still puddles of stale, gray water on the floor. Once inside, Fran saw that the room was deeper than could be seen from the hall no matter how open the door was. There was a row of six stalls. Inside the first one a man stood between the toilet and the metal wall between stalls and energetically masturbated. As his inflamed eyes rose to meet hers, she turned away.

"Maaama!"

She found Walter on the floor of the last stall, and hesitated for the briefest of moments, struck into stone by the sight of her son lying huddled next to the toilet, clutching his chest and stomach. The floor was wet and his pajama bottoms, which were bunched around his ankles, were soaked. Most of his top was soaked, too. Walter's eyes were closed and he was shivering. His hair was wet and sticking to his face, which was dirty with tears, sweat, filth, and stubble. "Walter," she cried in horror, and then started to sob.

Fran swallowed her sobs and went to her son, knelt beside the toilet and squeezed her arms around his wet shoulders, trying to cradle his head. Using all her strength she managed to lift him to a sitting position. Then she stroked his head and cleared the matted hair from his face.

"Maaama!" Walter sobbed.

"I'm here, Walter. I'm here."

"I hurt, Mama."

Feeling new strength, Fran moved him out from next to the toilet, sat on the wet floor herself, and cradled her son across her lap, holding his limp, tortured body close to her own, touching her head to his and rocking as she kissed his forehead.

This was the sight that arrested Dr. Lester as he came into the bathroom. Fran did not look up at him, but squeezed her son tighter as she rocked and the choking sobs broke inside her like stormswept waves.

[2]

Dazed, afraid to look at her watch for fear she had lived less than a lifetime in the last hour, Fran sat in her car and tried to swallow her anguish, tried to force it down to a place where it would not erupt on her and render her unable to negotiate the steps required to get her safely home.

The psych techs had come and taken Walter away, and Lester had offered to give her a sedative as he assured her that Walter was "just fine and dandy." She had wanted to drag her son out of the hospital and into her car and kidnap him—and it would be kidnapping, because legally he was not hers anymore. He was a child of the county. But the county had done this to him. The county was an abusive parent. And the county was stingy, whereas Fran would give her lifeblood to. . .

To do what? she asked herself in the car. To make him well? To make him better? Such considerations had been swept totally out of reach, if not over the past years, then certainly in the past hour.

To keep him alive.

To keep him from suffering.

Fran knew she would have to not cry if she were to make it home, but the sobs were coming now, anyway, and she couldn't stop them. Her dress still reeked of the awful smells of the bathroom. Walter had reeked of that same stink, and she knew the horror would never even begin to diminish until she got the stink out of the clothes . . . and now, she supposed, the car, too. The realization was too much for Fran, and she rested her head on the steering wheel and gave in again to the sobs.

At first she didn't hear the rapping on the window. But then she did. Her eyes were closed, and in the moment before she opened them she thought maybe it was Dr. Lester come out to apologize or tell her it was all a mistake and Walter would be moved some-where—or that he could even come home with her.

But it wasn't Dr. Lester. It was a woman about Fran's age wearing a round red hat with nylon lace, which was pinned up in her tightly styled gray hair. She had a kindly face, and she looked concerned.

Fran rolled down the window.

"Are you all right, dear?"

Fran wiped her eyes and nodded.

"Please forgive me, but . . . do you have a child in the hospital?"

Fran nodded again, felt another sob coming behind the admission.

"Well, I do, too. My son has been here for almost ten years. I don't know what you've just seen, exactly, but . . . well, we've all been through a lot. . . ." The woman examined Fran. "Are you okay?"

Fran nodded.

"My name is Anita Sansone. Look, I belong to a group of people who all have children or relatives in this hospital. Here, take this." She handed a card through the window. "That has my phone number. You can call me any time. We have a meeting coming up in just two weeks. You're invited."

Fran noticed that the woman's hand was extended through the window. Without thinking, she reached up and allowed the woman's hand to surround hers. She wanted to cry again. When she looked up into the other woman's eyes she saw that it was all right, that she was expecting her to, and that it was a good thing. So Fran rested her forehead on the woman's hand and let the waves wash her away again.

"You're okay," Anita said. "You're going to make it just fine. You know, we cry sometimes at our meetings." She took a deep breath, and as she stroked Fran's head gently with her other hand, she looked back at the hospital. "But we do some other things, too."

Fran heard this, despite the squall raking through her, and felt the other mother's hand tighten with confidence around her own. At that moment, she decided nothing was going to get in the way of her attending that meeting.

7

[1]

We have not progressed so far from the days of burning witches as we think we have.

During the latter half of the nineteenth century, the widespread construction of state mental hospitals resulted in a steady growth in the number of patients within them, a growth which began to rise dramatically toward the end of the century. Between 1890 and 1958, the number of hospitalized mentally ill rose from just under 100,000 to over 500,000. Then the Great Catastrophe occurred.

The Great Catastrophe began in the late fifties and early sixties with the community placement myth—the idea that the mentally ill were sick because of bad surroundings and could become well by absorbing sanity from a sane environment. Deinstitutionalization began with a denial of medical facts: the problem was that the mentally ill were warehoused in state hospitals, and all you had to do was get them out of the hospitals and the entire problem of mental illness would go away.

The plan was to farm out their care to community mental health centers. Get them out into the community, where they will lose the stigma of hospitalization.

Unfortunately, the money to fulfill these promises didn't follow the good intentions. Only about one-fifth as many community mental health centers were built as were supposed to be built. Centers were understaffed and underfunded, and though some fulfilled the promise of effective, compassionate care, most soon found they could not even begin to handle the seriously ill patients. So they focused their resources on a more comfortable and profitable clientele, the "worried well," middle-class people with mostly neurotic problems.

In two decades, most of the progress of the prior 150 years in organizing public care for the mentally ill was dismantled. By 1980, there were only about 100,000 people in state mental hospitals. That's a drop of 400,000 in only twenty-two years. Some of the original half million people in mental hospitals died, but they were more than replaced by new cases. The population eligible for hospital-level care was growing during those twenty-two years, not declining.

As a result, a great tide of chronic mentally ill washed over the community, and the entire system of care was thrown into a disarray from which it never recovered. As the eighties ended and the last decade of the twentieth century began, the availability and level of mental health services varied greatly from state to state and from county to county within the same state. There was no central, fixed point of reference or responsibility, no organized system of care for the sickest, least able to help themselves members of society. Patients wandered from one facility to another. Information was rarely shared among facilities—in fact, there were legal barriers to such unified record keeping. Money was scarce for housing, care, and other services, and there were few incentives to use funds efficiently. Instead, there was a proliferation of inefficient bureaucracies—cottage industries of care. The net profit on this venture was one million adult schizophrenics, more than half the total, none of whom were receiving professional care for their illness.

The Great Catastrophe created an army of misery, a refugee population roaming around the country, displaced victims of the ongoing war to liberate the mental hospitals. They were displaced by decisions which the society seemed to have made purposefully and deliberately. They were disenfranchised by virtue of their illness and by their inability to help themselves. There were more mentally ill people in jails and prisons than there were in mental hospitals.

During his waking hours, Alex Greco was haunted by these musings. He could not escape them, because the state hospital was the center ring in this circus of agony. In that ring were some of the most advanced arts that medical science could produce. At the same time, much that went on had changed little since medieval times.

Bedloe was now a poor stepchild of the state, an unwanted orphan. In 1962, its patient population was at its peak of over five thousand. Over the next two decades, the patient population was reduced to one thousand.

So why, Alex asked himself, was Bedloe the center ring? The hospital was a relic fort. Despite the massiveness of it, the sheer ambition of its original intentions, the hospital was now nothing but a rickety pier set up in a stormy sea from which they assumed, foolishly, that the concentration of resources could get a foothold in the battle.

Maybe that was why the hospital had endured. Perhaps the focus of so much misery and illness in one spot meant something in the flow of things, meant that because we had assembled our forces here, and brought with us not only those whom the Enemy had already taken, but a few who were still straddling the line, that the Enemy would be forced to come here, to attack here, to meet us here, and that whatever was learned about defeating the Enemy could be taken to other fronts.

But Alex knew that was not what was happening. How could you claim any kind of progress at all, regardless of what you knew, if more than half of the victims were receiving no care at all?

Alex knew Bedloe State Hospital was simultaneously hell and haven, dungeon and sanctuary. Yet he could not bring himself to think of it as a cave of unrelenting misery. Within those same walls were patience, compassion, courage, charity, and love. True, the confounding absurdities of the bureaucratic system frustrated the best efforts and intentions of the staff—but it was also a place where those efforts were sometimes victorious.

Lily Speere, the waif Alex had seen in the Receiving Unit in January, had returned to Bedloe. In February her father had died of a massive coronary. Two weeks later, a despondent Lily ignored the aspirin she had used in her New Year's flirtation with suicide and chose, instead, the antidepressants that had been prescribed for her grieving mother. Alex was determined that Bedloe would be a sanctuary for Lily, that her life would be saved here. He assigned her to Wilson Cottage and Doc.

Alex called Doc's extension. One ring. Two rings. Three rings. Four rings. Alex's heart sank. He knew that when Doc was on the ward the phone was always answered before the fourth ring.

Finally, Wendy answered the phone. She informed Alex that Doc had just left for the day.

Alex hung up the phone and took a deep breath which he quickly let out with a sigh. He would have to make it on his own, without a few minutes with Doc to reestablish a perspective that allowed him to see the world as a place where things happened, some of which were god-awful tragic and some of which were funny and some of which were both—but all of which were absolutely fascinating and worthy of appreciation.

There was a firm knock on Alex's door, which was already open just enough for Doc to poke in his head.

"Is this bar still open?" Doc whispered.

"This bar is always open," Alex said with genuine cheer. Doc was already halfway to the leather chairs across from the desk.

"I had a woman come this week, new patient." Doc always started this way, with a minimum of introductions, dispensing with formalities. "NGI. Not Guilty—Insane. Ethel Flynn." Doc paused for a moment, waiting.

"Shot her husband," Alex said. "I saw her records."

Doc nodded. "I let Rosey interview her," Doc said. "I went in with him, but tried to keep my mouth shut."

"Tried?" Alex picked up on the hint right away, knowing it was Doc's cue for the story.

"Ethel had steadfastly denied shooting her husband. I told Rosey that we had a choice with this woman. We could either let her vegetate here, or we could try to help her a bit. If we wanted to help her, the first step was getting her to confess to shooting her husband."

Alex nodded, already smiling in anticipation.

Doc caught the smile and returned it with one of his own as he went on. "So Ethel comes in and—she's not an unattractive woman, I might add—and Rosey is ready with the goods. 'Mrs. Flynn,' he says, 'why did you shoot your husband?'

" 'I didn't shoot the sonofabitch,' she says.

"But Rosey was ready with the evidence: 'Look, Mrs. Flynn, here's the police report. Here is the court transcript of your husband's testimony. All the evidence is right here. Of course you shot your husband!' "

Doc leaned over and gently placed his palm down on Alex's desk. Then he want on, speaking softly, "Ethel shook her head. 'I couldn't have shot my husband,' she said. 'In the first place there wasn't a gun in the house.' " Doc solemnly slapped the desk for emphasis, then raised his hand again. " 'In the second place the bullets wouldn't fit the gun.' "

The hand came down again, a little harder. " 'And in the third place he was too far away to hit!' "

As Doc slammed the desk again, he exploded in a coughing fit of laughter. Alex giggled mischievously. Through the giggling, he asked Doc, "What'd you do?"

"What do you think? Exactly what I'm doing now. I burst out laughing! And so did Ethel!" With that admission, Doc was bent over in another spasm. When he was almost recovered, he went on, "You've got to enjoy someone who talks like that."

Alex had tears in his eyes, yet he managed to hiccup out a question, "What did the resident do?"

Doc smiled broadly, his eyes twinkling, and said, "Rosey was struck dumb. I think he wanted to cry. Or disappear."

Alex nodded.

"I told Ethel we'd see her again in a day or two. She kind of smiled, too. I think she'll come around just fine."

"How about Rosey?

Doc smiled. "As I always say, not everyone gets well. But just about everyone can get better. Rosey may put this adage to the test, though."

Alex nodded. From what he's seen of young Dr. Rose, he suspected the man was too sensitive, too vulnerable for a place like Bedloe.

"He's a good kid, a good and caring physician," Doc went on. "But I think he may have a problem with the boundaries between doctor and patient. He wants to be friends with his patients."

"Buddies."

Doc nodded. There was a moment of silence while the two men let the subject of Rosey drift away. Neither wanted to take it any further right then, since that would mean getting too close to discussing what they sensed was the real problem: Steven Rose had a curiosity about the mind, but not a genuine enthusiasm for psychiatry. He often seemed repulsed by the very methods and procedures the two older, experienced physicians held as absolute requirements for the job. At times he even appeared to be disgusted by what he perceived as their coarseness.

But they also knew that he could grow out of that. Alex and Doc had—as a matter of survival.

Worse, however, was Alex's suspicion that Rose's lack of enthusiasm for psychiatry appeared to be shared by a great many young physicians. Psychiatric residencies were dropping off. Some doctors said it was because psychiatrists were, on average, among the lowest-earning physicians. Others said it was because psychiatry was historically the most liberal of the specialties, and we were living in a conservative era. Still others said it was because psychiatry was a stalking horse for all the bad things that were about to happen in medicine. "Can't blame him. What young physician," Alex asked, "would volunteer to be cannon fodder for the coming upheavals?"

"Not me," Doc declared, unconvincingly.

After the pause, Alex asked, "How's Lily Speere?"

Doc nodded. "She's coming along nicely. I think the meds are working. She had enough spirit to argue with Wendy yesterday."

Alex smiled. "Good. I wasn't sure antidepressants would work with her."

"Ask Wendy. She's the expert on medications. And she's convinced Lily's just biding her time."

"What do you think, Doc?"

Doc stood up. "I think I'm going on vacation, Doctor. Be gone a week."

Alex understood. Doc felt Lily Speere would be fine and didn't want to talk about her anymore.

Alex nodded. "Heading for the shore again?"

Doc paused and a philosophical glaze came over his eyes. "I personally hate the feel of sand between my toes. But as long as Milly owns the car, I guess I'll go wherever she wants to drive me." Then Doc resumed walking toward the door.

"If you run into any medical waste from Bedloe, don't let on you recognize it."

Doc waved without turning and was gone.

Alex sighed deeply. He was proud to be a psychiatrist again. There was something restorative in his contact with Doc. Whatever it was about Bedloe that confounded his sense of being a good physician, Doc was immune to it. He was so purely identified with being a physician and a psychiatrist that none of the extraneous matters distracted him. For Alex, spending a few moments with Doc was like looking through a window at what psychiatry really was.

He could go home now.

8 _____

Wendy held the ring of keys still and carefully selected the one she knew was right. She checked the hall in both directions to make sure no one was watching, then slipped the key into the lock, turned it, and opened the door in as fluid a motion as its machinery would allow. She closed the door behind her quickly, but quietly, and locked it.

She was in a small, empty reception office. The single gray state-issue iron desk was bare except for a decrepit table lamp. The room felt cold. Sensing there was someone present, Wendy stopped before opening the inner door next to the desk. Her body tensed.

"Bert? That you?"

There was no answer from the next room, a large examining room, also unused. She was certain now that someone was in the room. She gave the door a slight push with her foot, enough to open it another foot . . . if it just . . . kept going . . . then she would be able to see.

"C'mere, baby."

Wendy sighed. "Bert, fruck-a-duck!" For a moment she wanted to be angry or defiant, but when she pushed open the door and saw his slender body in the gray light of the vacant examination room, she wanted to collapse into his arms.

When she saw the flower he held out to her, she did just that.

"C'mere, baby," Bert said again, after she was tight in his embrace. He kissed her forehead, then worked down to her eyes and the side of her face.

"Oh, Bert."

Wendy felt herself weaken as Bert's arms tightened around her and seemed to support her. She felt his legs slip under hers to lift and do the work as his hands caressed her back. He seemed to be gathering her up, pulling her on top of him even while they stood. Bert seemed to expand as his arms enveloped her, and she shrank into him. He bit at her lips and lifted her up and over to the green vinyl sofa in the corner of the room. Wendy felt the life in him all around her, tugging at her clothes, fumbling with his own, but also in his breath and his odor and in the electricity of his skin, which sent shivers through her skin into her own center. This was just what she needed, a big dose of life. The thought floated into her head, like a long-suppressed conviction: This is what life is.

"Bert, you are one hot man." Wendy squirmed under him and smiled. The only answer he gave her was to let one of his heavy, damp breaths sag into a moan.

Wendy retreated into herself again. She knew Bert would take a few minutes to come back into the world anyway. The smell rising off their bodies caught her suddenly, a sweet smell, but also musty. She knew it wasn't perfume. It was the life smell, the vague honeystink left over after sex.

Wendy knew why it struck her so. It was so much like the odor of the leaves in the woods, in the places where you dug below the surface to where the leaves were black and crumbling into the dirt, warm with the burning of decay, which, after all, was a kind of life, too.

9

Lily Speere lay on her bed and frowned at the thought of the old man doctor who had abandoned her.

Doc says this and Doc says that and Doc left me. So who needs him? So who needs anybody? So who needs Lily?

Just when things were getting good he goes away.

It was a bad thing to do. But not as bad as what Lily can do. No matter how bad the things they do are, Lily can do something worse.

Oh, it is just too, too sad. And Lily is too, too mad.

Lily felt the anguish like a heavy weight growing inside her and pressing. Now it was in her head, a pulsing knot of vulnerability and outrage. But it would move down to her chest and try to block off her air, squeeze her heart until it couldn't beat anymore.

Lily doesn't care. Why should Lily care?

Well, I'll just show Doc. I don't care. Why should I care?

Lily reached under her mattress and pressed the springs apart until she could withdraw the little bundle. She put the bundle on her chest and watched her breath make it go up and down and up and down like a boat on a stormy sea.

I can sink this boat. I can sink this whole damn sea.

Just watch me. I am Poseidon. I am the god of the sea. All knowing comes from little old me. My snot is the stuff of life, and the color of angels' eyes.

Lily slowly, ceremoniously unwrapped the handkerchief bundle, lifting one flap after another until the green shard of glass lay on the cloth like a jewel.

Beautiful bad, bad, bad. Lily is beautiful bad.

Old damn Doc left me, so here's for you, old damn Doc. And here's for me.

Lily picked up the shard, careful to avoid the sharp edge, where little flakes of fresh glass still clung and sparkled.

This is our body. This is our blood, which shall be shed for us.

Lily lifted the shard over her until it captured the lightbulb on the ceiling and took on for her the resplendence of a holy sacrificial knife.

I am sinking into a big black hole and it feels so cool and comfortable down here. I am safe at last.

Lily arm's seemed to grow as she fell away from the shard, deeper and deeper away.

Oh, valiant knight, come and close my eyes with your kiss. Come and do this thing. Save me.

Lily's arms shortened now, as the shard descended.

It hurts so beautiful bad.

Lily held the shard with both hands, as a priest grips the Host, and brought it to her lips and gave it a long, final kiss.

The blade is already warm with my life.

She held the shard in front of her face, manipulating it with her fingers until it was rotated in just the right attitude as she brought it down to the base of her neck.

It hurts so beautiful bad.

With a jerk she dug the sharp edge into the base of her neck.

My blood is cool.

She pressed the shard edge deeper, feeling the blood lubricate it as it slid into and across her throat, and she gave in to a gurgling cry as the last strength in her arms drew it from one end to the other and then back again.

Father! Oh, bad, bad, bad!

10

A few days after Doc went on vacation, Alex received a call from the Family Organization. Anita Sansone asked him if he would attend their upcoming meeting, and he accepted the invitation.

Alex had heard about the incident involving Fran Channing in D-7. Late in February, in a meeting with Sam Akbar about administrative matters, he had brought up the need for a thorough reform of the unit. Akbar had not only crudely dismissed Alex's concern by waving his hand and barking, "This kind of crap goes on all the time!" but he had, to Alex's astonishment, swept away all of the administrative points, too. "The answer is no to everything, Alex."

Alex was not so much demoralized by Akbar himself as by the knowledge that the superintendent was just a crude representation of the state's attitude. Akbar's appointment had come, after all, from the highest levels of the state department of mental health.

[2]

The Family Organization was part of a nationwide alliance that was already over 130,000 strong, growing rapidly, and well on its way to becoming a political power locally, in state legislatures, and nationally. Chapters of the organization could be extremely helpful, persuasive, or, if necessary, bothersome to hospital and state mental-health administrations. Yet most of their gains, Alex knew, had been won by the sheer persistence of the middle-class outrage fueled from the depths of their anguish.

From past experience, Alex knew that these parents seemed to understand the system as well as he did. Maybe that was because fighting the system was their life, because the survival of their loved ones was at stake. They had learned long ago that this was no consumer issue, not a question of whether too many tonsillectomies were performed. This was the life or death of their children. In the Organization literature Alex had read that members sometimes feared for their children's lives if they spoke out too vehemently. The stories told of children transferred to more restrictive units, or provoked into assaultive behavior if the parents became too vocal in their criticism.

Since Bedloe State Hospital drew its patients from an area of several thousand square miles, the Family Organization meetings were held in a more or less central location, a town half an hour away from the hospital. Alex enjoyed the drive, but felt a twist in his gut when he saw the church where the meeting was being held. He pulled into the lot and parked at the far end. As he got out of the car and walked toward a group of people milling around in the floodlit entrance to the church basement, he heard laughter.

"Oh, you must be Dr. Greco. Welcome!" a short, smartly dressed woman said with a warmth that Alex had not expected. She took his hand and squeezed it. "I'm Anita Sansone. I invited you to come tonight. I'm so glad you could make it." She turned to the others. "Let me introduce you."

To Alex's surprise the introductions went smoothly, smiles all around. Only one woman in the group seemed to have trouble smiling. She had blond hair and her eyes seemed to be brimming with emotion. She was a person, Alex could tell, who felt everything very intensely. He knew he had seen her somewhere before . . . or heard her voice. Of course—she was the mother of the schizophrenic boy in D-7, Walter Channing. Alex had seen her and her son entering the Receiving Unit two months ago.

"Mrs. Channing . . ."

She turned to Alex, unable to erase the pain from her face, but trying to smile.

"I'm Alex Greco."

"Yes . . ."

Suddenly, Alex felt the awkwardness, too. This woman's son was a patient in his hospital. She should be asking him about Walter's condition, but she wasn't. He decided to try to put them both at ease. "Walter is doing fine."

Fran nodded. "Thank you, Dr. Greco. I spoke to Walter on the phone yesterday."

Alex could tell she wanted to say more. The whole group was making a special effort to be nice to him, to make him feel comfortable. Yet he couldn't be the charming Hollywood doctor. I cannot be graceful in this, he thought. Alex felt his awkwardness, felt the bulk of his body as something to be steered, managed, sailed on a zigzag course between these people and their horrific experiences and his own need to be a professional. *We're doing what we can, or less than we can. But this is war, remember that. People's lives are smashed.*

As Alex moved among the family members, and a few politely expressed their frustrations with the hospital, it seemed clear they knew that superintendent Sam Akbar was the sore point. They were frustrated that, under Akbar, the hospital was closed to them for all but the briefest visits with their children. Alex knew why. In a conversation about the organization, Sam had said to Alex that the parents could really "gum up the works." "They think they can run the place once you let them in," he had confided. Sam had refused the Organization permission to contact other relatives of patients at Bedloe, or even to leave pamphlets notifying family members of where they could obtain support in their struggles.

But Alex could tell that they also knew that Akbar was not the sole reason for conditions at Bedloe, that there were problems and problem people at every level.

The group of three or four dozen filed into the neat, carpeted basement and sat in folding chairs arranged in close rows in front of the podium.

After briefly getting through the incidentals and introducing Alex for the benefit of members who hadn't met him personally, Anita Sansone introduced a tall man about Alex's age, neatly dressed in a gray suit. Alex could see the heat in this man's eyes as he grabbed the edge of the podium. With his first sentence, the man routed the nervous protocol that had reigned since Alex's arrival:

"My daughter was at Bedloe and she was raped, and we still had to go to court to get her out of there. And we couldn't. . . ." His voice started to break. "See, when she first got sick, about ten years ago, when she was sixteen, well, I had us covered, health insurance. But once she was diagnosed schizophrenic, the insurance company said they'd pay 50 percent for one year of treatment and that was it. Sure enough, a year later they canceled her coverage.

"She had gotten better after six months of treatment, and lived at home for awhile, but then she got sick again and we didn't know what to do. All we could do is let the county take over. So when she was raped, they told us we didn't have anything to say about her care anymore."

The man's chest seemed to swell and his chin rose and set firmly. "We got together with the county man, and he was a good guy. He sent an ambulance for her. And she was back in the county facility that night. He said she wouldn't ever have to go back to Bedloe again. We slept the whole night for the first time in months that night.

"It gets so you don't think about things like having her home again, for good I mean, or having her well, but just having her nearby and not on the streets or being hurt, just . . ." His voice broke up and his head hung low. "Well, that didn't last. We visited her every day. Every day. Brought her candy bunny rabbits. Funny, when she was three she was crazy about candy bunny rabbits. Now she's . . . twenty-six and a candy bunny rabbit is about the only thing that makes her smile. . . .

"But two days later, God, it was only about three hours after I left her side at the county center, she called us on the phone and said, 'Daddy, they took me back, they took me back! Don't let them keep me here, please don't let them. . . .' " Then the man's voice broke and he stopped talking while he fought for control.

He looked up but tried not to let his eyes make contact with another person. "They had come for her that afternoon, not half an hour after we left her, and taken her back to Bedloe. Nobody knew about it, not even the county man. It was the hospital people did it."

No, Alex thought to himself, the county made those decisions, always protecting itself from the potentially costly effects of compassion. When the county wants them back, they get them back, regardless of what the hospital wants. Or vice versa, if they don't want them back. This apparently had been one of the vice versas, in which a county bureaucrat somewhere had added up a column of figures and decided the young woman's care would be cheaper at Bedloe than at the county facility. Sometimes the counties had beds at the hospital that were paid up in advance and had to be used.

An auburn-haired woman of about forty-five got up before the group. Alex could tell she was making a special effort to keep her chin straight out in front of her face, and the effect was one of forced strength. He did it himself sometimes.

"My son first became ill when he was nineteen." She dropped her chin for a moment, struggling with her nervousness. "During his first hospitalization he was kept in seclusion for more than two weeks. We were not allowed to see him. The only person he was allowed to see was his therapist, who brought him his food three times a day." Her face dropped again. Her voice cracked when she began speaking again. "When he came out of that hospital—it was a private hospital, by the way—he was much, much worse. He looked like a zombie. He didn't even recognize his father and me." Her chin dropped all the way to her chest now as she fought for control. "That was only the beginning."

I know these stories, Alex thought. I hear them every day, I live them. I can open any file and find this horror.

A short, stocky woman of about fifty-five, who seemed overdressed in a sequined shift, took the microphone in her hands, which were nervously searching for something more to hold, and said, "My daughter has been ill for twenty-one years. She has been in about sixteen different hospitals and various mental health facilities. And she's lived on the streets. Right now she's on the streets. I pray God she's taken care of. I don't know where she is. It's been four months since I've heard from her." The woman could not go on, or was done anyway, and another woman helped her get back to her seat.

A fortyish woman in a blue suit went to the podium next. She pinched the bridge of her nose and seemed to be concentrating very hard. Then she looked up at the group.

"My name is Rebecca Grossman. . . . I sometimes ask myself how will I get to sleep tonight? How will there ever be sleeping again? Then I tell myself there will be, there will have to be. I need the rest."

Rebecca took a deep breath. "My husband Michael died five years ago. At night sometimes when I feel alone I sit in his big leather chair by the bookcase under his reading lamp. There's a little table there with his pipes on it. I've kept everything just the way he liked it. And I pick up one of the pipes and hold it close enough to my face to smell the tobacco." Her voice cracked a little, but when a woman from the audience rose and started toward her, Rebecca shook her head and smiled. The woman sat down.

"I have my son Todd's catcher's mitt from when he was in Little League. I have a few old pairs of his shoes. I have lots of photographs. I have his bedroom just the way he liked it. But that's all I have of my son. I don't know where he is, whether he's living or dead. I want to tell you the story.

"Todd walked and spoke in sentences at eleven months. We kept a list of his words on the refrigerator and had to buy more magnetic letters and use the stove and the dishwasher door." Rebecca's right hand clenched into a fist and slammed into the other one.

"When he was two he seemed to have instant recall of the commercials on TV. . . ."

Alex's head began to buzz, he'd been through this story so many times before. He knew what was coming. The entire room did.

"He hated math class in school because it went too slow for him. When Michael, my husband, taught him to ride the bicycle, he held on to the back of the seat—but Todd took off all by himself, leaving his father screaming and chasing after him. We have that one"— her voice cracked—"on film. It's so funny."

"Go on, Rebecca. You're okay. We're with you, honey."

Alex found himself unable to observe this scene from any kind of comfortable professional distance. The people in the room seemed to draw around Rebecca, leaning forward from their seats. Alex was amazed that all this misfortune and pain had not produced mean-spirited people. On the contrary, they seemed most generous with the human commodities life had withheld from them.

"Todd's first breakdown, if you can call it that, came one morning when he was barely sixteen. He was late getting down to breakfast—which wasn't all that unusual. But this time he just didn't respond to my calls. 'He's probably just sick,' Michael said as he rushed out the door, 'call me and let me know.'

"Well, when I went up, I found Todd just lying there, like a dead person, staring at the ceiling. I spoke to him, touched him—oh, he was cold!—and all he said was he was heavy as the world. That's all he would say. He didn't even seem to know I was there, or who I was.

"I called my husband, and he came right home. 'I don't know what to do, Michael,' I said. He didn't know what to do either, except to talk to Todd. But the boy just started shaking and chattering his teeth. . . ."

She struggled for control, hoisting her head by tightening the muscles of her neck and back, setting her jaw straight. "And now, seven years later, I'm convinced that no one really knows what to do, and that the most we can hope for in this world is for people to admit they don't know what to do, even though they're pretending to know."

Alex knew all about the word "hope." It was used frequently in the books and pamphlets Rebecca and her husband would have read, along with all the people in the room, including himself. It was a word used in medical journals, although sparingly, self-consciously. The word would have been spoken by the professionals who examined Todd, by clergy, by friends and other family members who obviously didn't know what else to say.

"Michael, after two years of trying, just gave up. He died. What ate him up was the way Todd's good days were as good as the good days had ever been, so good that we started to believe the bad days were gone forever, or that they were some kind of awful nightmare. But then would come the bad days, and they could be so bad that you had to wonder whether the good days were just part of the torture."

Rebecca's husband had run out of hope, or whatever fundamental thought we hold on to in order to keep alive. Alex wondered whether it was we who let go of the fundamental thought, or the Thought who let go of us.

But there was something in the woman's demeanor, the way her body would not let itself sag for more than a second before it responded with a tremendous effort to right itself, that told Alex she understood how her husband had let go. Expired. In her terror at being left alone, she most likely had felt a moment's anger, and then a taste of the same appetite for oblivion. But she had too much to do, too much immediate anguish, so she allowed herself only a brief paroxysm of grief at the loss of her husband.

"I felt like a stone fist had been slammed into the goodness of our lives. I didn't know what to do. My mind just spun around. To me, it seemed that life had gone crazy, not just my Todd, but life itself. I thought Todd's illness was the worst thing that could happen, but it wasn't. I thought Michael's death was the worst, but it wasn't. I thought my life couldn't possibly become more painful or difficult. I was mistaken."

Here's where we begin to understand that nothing holds, Alex knew; not the family, not the center of her life, not the fringes, not any of the connections in between. Nothing holds.

"My health insurance company reduced my coverage for Todd three times in the first year. On the day before his eighteenth birthday I received a letter informing me that his coverage would be terminated as of his birthday. There was nothing to be done. My attorney, the best man at our wedding, a good family friend, told me that fighting the insurance company would take years and Todd would spend those years in public hospitals anyway. My legal expenses would be unrecoverable, even if we won. And most likely we would not win.

"Then he said, 'Rebecca, it's not just the insurance company we're up against. It's history.' He said that, and I'll never forget it. 'Medical care is just getting more and more expensive and, frankly, nobody has enough money to pay for it. Not you, not me, not the government, not the insurance companies. The only answer is just to cut off certain areas of care. We're starting with mental illness, because, frankly—I'm sorry to be so blunt—nobody cares about the mentally ill. They have no effective lobby. Next will be people with AIDS. The attitude is, they're all homosexuals and drug addicts anyway, so who cares? Then old people—we're already seeing that. Medicare doesn't cover everything. And the things it does cover, well, you had better just be able to find a doctor and a hospital who will fix you up for the amount of money Medicare's willing to pay.'

"Then he told me about his aunt who had just died. She was put out of the hospital two days after her operation. Two days! An eighty-one-year-old woman. 'It's history, Rebecca,' he said. 'We're living in a stingy, mean, brutish time. A sorry, shameful time.'

"Then he apologized for getting so emotional and said his best advice was to get Todd into the county system of care as fast as possible. Which is what I did.

"And I went to therapy, myself. The same insurance that dropped my son would still pay for ten sessions of therapy for me, so I went for it."

"Good for you, Becky!" a woman sitting next to Fran Channing shouted. A few people started to applaud.

" 'You are a separate being,' my therapist advised me. My life is distinct from Todd's. This is what I learned in therapy. I may feel pain for my son, but I am not connected to him by nerves or blood vessels."

Alex listened to the litany taught to Rebecca by the therapist, which she was to chant to herself every time she felt overwhelmed: "I have a job. I earn money and take care of myself. I live in my house. I buy food and prepare it for myself. I have friends who love me—"

"Yes, you certainly do, Becky," Fran said.

"We love you, Rebecca," another woman said, as applause scattered through the room.

Rebecca smiled and nodded, and then continued, "I live in a world where good things and bad things happen. I can make it through. Todd is my son. I love Todd. Todd loves me. Todd is ill. I do all I can for Todd. His illness is not my illness. I do all I can for Todd. I do. . ."

It was not working, and Alex knew from experience that it didn't work. It was not holding back the pain because the loss was just too great. When a chasm that immense opens in a life, it pulls the strongest of us into it.

Alex closed his eyes and saw the rest of the story as Rebecca described it. There is a way people say good-bye when they know it may be the last time, when they know there is something irretrievable in their lives that is passing and they are acknowledging it as completely as their capacity for loss will allow. Such a time was the night Rebecca Grossman said goodbye to her son at midnight in the drizzle outside the county mental health center, where the psychologist in charge insisted she hand him over to attendants. It was Todd's seventeenth admission in three years.

Images of the pathetic scene trickled into Alex's consciousness with Rebecca Grossman's words. He saw the parking lot polished black by the rain, the sick boy's curly hair hanging down all wet and dripping, the men standing at the doorway impatient and ignorant of the mother's need to say something or do something to help her son go, the blank look in Todd's eyes, the way his mouth just hung half open, the way he just stood there and let the rain come down on him.

Then, and now, the mother was not able to stem the flood of tears. Tortured by the scene, by her complete failure to do anything for Todd, by having to give her sick little boy over to strangers, she bitterly lost all resistance to sorrow.

Because that was the last time she had seen her son. Two weeks later, Todd's social worker at the center had called and asked how Todd was doing at home with his new medications.

Rebecca had asked what he meant, she hadn't seen Todd in two weeks because the staff had told her they thought it would be better this time if she didn't visit or call for at least a month.

Alex felt the pit in his gut start to burn. He knew what was coming.

There had been a silence on the line. Then the social worker had said he would call back—but Rebecca told him to wait, what was going on?

Another silence. The social worker cleared his throat. "Mrs. Grossman, Todd was discharged. I . . . I'll get back to you. Thank you," he said and hung up.

Alex opened his eyes to escape, but there was the mother, right in front of him, devastated but determined to finish her story.

"Several frantic calls later," Rebecca said, "I learned that after a week the center had discharged Todd in the middle of the night with a month's worth of medications and put him into a taxicab. He never arrived home. No one had any idea where he was. That was a month ago."

At that moment, Rebecca started to cry again, clearly forgetting everything her therapist had taught her about being a separate being able to feel joy. "All I do now is concentrate in my heart, trying to feel the life of my little boy out in the world somewhere, just to sense that he is alive."

Everyone in the room sat in silence, letting Rebecca's story find the places in their hearts where their own stories were remembered, letting Rebecca set free her pain and letting her pain find theirs and liberate their sorrow.

But there is an unending supply of sorrow, Alex thought. And the heart must make room for more, or else it will burst. That is what is going on here. As he listened to Rebecca's story, the rush of fresh remembrance brought a softening to the tightness in his chest, and Alex felt a ball of emotion rising in him. He clenched his fists tightly in his lap and forced his lips against one another. Then, when he knew he had forced it down, he reached up and squeezed his eyes and the bridge of his nose. Alex had long ago run out of explanations for every horror. He knew somewhere someone was lamenting this way for Deborah Smith, the murdered patient found at Poe Lake, and all the other lost children.

And then Rebecca was finished, and she came back and sat down at the end of the same aisle Alex was in. He shuddered.

The next person to get up was a man about Alex's age, but wearing a black T-shirt that showed his muscular arms. Alex thought he saw a Corps tattoo on one arm and so looked him over closely. Yes, he could have been a Marine. He still wore his hair as short as a barber could make it and still call it a haircut rather than a shave.

The man cleared his throat. "My name, as most of you know already, is Albert. My daughter's been mentally ill since she was twenty-one. She's schizophrenic. She was in a different hospital every year for the first ten or eleven years or so. She lived on the streets for a time. She was abducted and raped. She got into drugs." Albert paused to take a deep breath and exhale some pain.

Albert went on. "My daughter is in a drug-rehab program now at the county facility. She lives at Mercy Board and Care, which many of you know about. It's an all right place." Albert looked around the room. "She's making progress."

A few people in the room applauded.

"She's . . ." Albert choked on his words. "She . . . she's still my little girl and . . . and I'm proud of her. She's a real fighter." Albert jerked his head to the side as if an invisible hand had slapped him, and as the room broke into applause, he bolted back to his seat.

As Alex watched the man thump back into his chair, he felt the swell rising in him, and he knew he was not going to be able to fight this one down. It was Alex's turn to bolt. He rose and nodded his excuse-mes as he made his way to the end of the aisle. He didn't want to take a chance on trying to say anything because there was no telling what was waiting in his throat.

He found out soon enough, in the men's room, which, thankfully, was empty. He closed his eyes to the mirror, jammed the faucet on full blast, and released his own torrent as he splashed water over his face. The stories in the other room had cast a spell on him, and he was fighting it with water and tears. He and the other parents were partners in despair. They all loved children who had been shanghaied into the dark realm.

Alex gagged on his own sorrow, for all he could see was his own child, growing up before his eyes and disappearing into a nightmare.

11 _____

A plan. That's what Carmen Greco needed, a plan. And she knew it, too.

That's why she had gone into the store and had come out with the pencils. You needed lots of pencils to write down a plan. Paper she had plenty of. She could use the blank edges of the newspapers she had lying around the house, piled on every table and chair. If she wrote nice and small she could fit all her plans right alongside the features and news stories. Nobody wrote small better than Carmen.

She would sharpen her pencils to a razor point with the paring knife.

The only problem there was you got lead all over the fruit when you sliced it.

No big deal.

1. Get pencils.

2. Throw away old plans.

3. Start over.

Full-page ads were the best, the ones with big pictures, because they usually had lots of blank space on the page and Carmen didn't have to write so small.

1. Get a new job.

The job at T-Mart wasn't working out. Carmen had found this real neat children's book and was sitting down reading it when she was supposed to be rearranging the shelves and the manager came by. She could tell from the way he spoke to her that her days were numbered, and, besides, he was a son of a bitch. The story was he abused his kids and his wife and beat the dog.

1. Write a letter to T-Mart home office about Frank.

2. Get severance pay.

3. Buy the children's book at T-Mart.

Carmen crossed out the last item.

3. Find out the title of the children's book.

4. Buy it.

5. Read the children's book.

A book like that could change your life, Carmen thought.

6. Change your life.

Nobody's life needed changing more than Carmen's, and she knew it, too.

7. Call Dad.

She crossed out item 7.

7. Call your father.

She crossed out item 7 again.

7. Call Dad, your father.

8. The psychiatrist.

12

March was an uncomfortable month for Alex. The tilting of the earth toward spring had a stirring, unsettling effect. The nights were still long and dark and cold, and Alex's dream still haunted him. But in the dreary sunless days a damp thawing was going on. The ground lay heavy and flat under the weight of melted snows. Spots of yellow-orange and purple here and there around the base of naked black trees gave notice that the earth was awakening. People were waking up, although some thought it was too soon to come out of their heavy clothes. Winter could still come back and show just how hard the earth could be frozen.

The mud of March froze and thawed and froze again . . . and finally dried as spring came and gave a deeper, more trustworthy blue to the sky. Even a surprise half-foot of snow during the last week of the month failed to dampen any more than a few early daffodils' enthusiasm for spring. Bedloe State Hospital decided it was time to put winter in the closet and go on. The grounds crew

95

made an appearance or two with rakes instead of snowshovels. New sheets of cardboard or plastic were installed by psych techs in broken windows which had never been repaired. A new rehab therapist in one of the adolescent wards began a car-washing service so her patients could earn money for excursions to the movies.

The handwriting of spring was in the sky. Flocks of birds swooped from bare tree to bare tree like the ghosts of leaves. This was enough for most people. Scarves and stiff coats were left in the closet, and necks were now free to turn and let the eyes see that the world was not a frigid tunnel from fireplace to furnace, but a huge soggy garden, growing all manner of things.

On warmer days, the earth gave up a sweet, musty aroma which to Alex was a promise as well as a reminder. In a few weeks the hospital grounds would be burgeoning with flowers and the wards with assaults and suicide attempts. Alex was aware that this could be interpreted as a natural rhythm, a dance whose steps were too deep and powerful to resist. But though his own life responded with excitement, he still wanted a better world.

As the vapors of Alex's restless discontent rose, he began a new painting. Convicted of witchcraft, three women were being burned at the stake.

As March's flirtations with spring gave way to April's love affair, Alex grew even more restless. He would open the window in his office a little bit wider every day and test the air for the scent of flowers. He would coax another five miles per hour out of the Lincoln on the way home, wanting to quickly put as much distance as he could between himself and the hospital. Finally, in midmonth there came that inevitable first day of deep, summer-like warmth and bright, unhesitant sunshine; the first day when the air was confidently sweet. It was a day to leave early.

Nearing home, Alex planned the rest of his day. In another few minutes he would pull into his driveway, swing through the white picket gate, hurry up the steps into the house, and change his clothes.

Then he and his wife Maria would go for a walk to the baseball field, and Alex would try to shake off the horrors of the day, not by talking about them, but by walking fast and making pointed observations about beautiful things he noticed along the walk. "Look at that bird's nest, wow!" Alex would exclaim when he spotted a tangle of straw and leaves high in the bare branches of an oak tree. "Look at that house, terrific!" Or, noticing something peculiar about the quality of the sky, he would squeeze Maria's hand and jab the index finger of his free hand skyward and pronounce, "That's just amazing!"

There was a comfort that came to Alex on these walks. The weight of his adult awareness seemed to drop away and in its place there arose a childlike ability to appreciate something as simple as a tree trunk shaped like a person's face. They always came back from the walks refreshed, and from that point on, the rest of the evening could be a near picture-perfect American family portrait. They sat down to dinner around a huge mahogany table with their daughter Stacy, eleven, and their son Anthony, nine, said a prayer, ate amidst chatter and announcements, cleared the table, and retired to the soft furniture of the living room for two hours or so of television. Sometime between 9:30 and 10:00 everyone went to bed.

But today, before Alex and Maria could get out the door, the phone rang. Alex looked at Maria, and then both turned their eyes away from each other and from the consideration of walking out without answering.

The call did not begin with the usual "Hi, Dad!" No pretense to normalcy at all: Alex answered the phone and heard only the long distance hiss . . . then the breathing . . . and then, just enough time after he realized who was at the other end, just enough time for the dread to have opened up a soft place in him, his daughter Carmen spoke, "Dad, I'm gonna go to jail 'cuz I got over a hundred parking tickets and they put a boot on my car and I hadda go in and they won't let me outa here unless I come up with the money."

Alex took a deep breath. There was not going to be any gradual sliding down tonight. No clumsy comic to warm up the audience. Just Blam, showtime! Put the psychiatrist in a box and saw it in half.

"Where are you?"

"Inna jail. Cop's right here, looking at me. I need a hundred dollars just to get outta here. Then I need six hundred and eighty-nine to get my car back. Dollars. Dad."

"Did you talk to Amy?" Amy was Carmen's maternal grandmother, a severe woman who had testified against Alex in the custody battle that accompanied his divorce. Amy had a great stake in denying her grandchild's illness, since Carmen was, almost to the most minute avenues of her brain's miswired circuitry, the identical map of her mother.

"Amy's gonna help. Amy's gonna help, Dad. She told me not to call you. She said you ought to help, you ought to care what happens to your daughter, and she said not to call you. I could use a couple hundred dollars here, Dad. I won't tell Amy."

Alex swallowed hard. "Carmen, let me talk to the desk sergeant."

"Sergeant? I dunno who the sergeant is. Look, I'm in this hallway and there's cops standing at the other end looking at me and they said I could make this call and I already talked to Amy and she said—"

"Carmen, let me talk to one of the cops. Tell one of the cops I want to talk to him. It's very important."

There was silence for a moment, then the sound of the receiver hitting the wall as it fell and dangled . . . then a few moments of silence . . . then Alex thought he could actually hear the phone being grasped, hear the fingers going around the handset and the handset lifted through the air . . . and hung up.

There had been an instant impulse to call back—but where?

He hung up the phone and his eyes immediately met Maria's. He turned away, then stared back into her eyes, his own eyes glaring with a determined fire he stoked from the inside: "Same old shit! Blah! Blah! Blah!"

"Do you want to go for a walk and talk about it?"

"Yeah, right!" Alex paced like a caged tiger who smells danger.

Maria prevailed over the confusion of his anguish. Alex was silent during the entire twenty minutes it took them to walk to the baseball field, which, at twilight, was lit up as if the World Series were being played. And he was silent as they began their regular circle of the field, where cardboard popcorn boxes discarded at the last game and soaked by the previous night's rain now sagged and collapsed. Alex kicked one that lay in his path.

This call from Carmen was relatively unremarkable. There had been hundreds like it over the years, and there would be hundreds more. There was nothing he could do to stop the calls, just as there was nothing he could do to plug the drain of enthusiasm and cheeriness that sometimes lightened his daughter's voice at the beginning. As the call progressed, the conversation became, against all the forces of his will and training, more and more disorganized, less a conversation between a father and daughter, less even one between a psychiatrist and a severely distraught patient. It finally became a raw struggle between his attempt to keep his daughter attached to some semblance of reason and the voracious maw that sucked her away.

"I am a four-star general in this war," Alex muttered. "My daughter has been taken prisoner . . . tortured . . . and the Enemy allows her, encourages her, to call me up in the throes of her agony."

But the Enemy was cunning and cruel, and struck closest to your heart, always.

[2]

Alex had met Carmen's mother at a dance during the first year of his residency, the year when all psychiatric residents believe that no one is really "crazy," but just in need of the kind of love and care that he was more than willing to give this wildly beautiful woman with the eyes that opened wide and saw so much. The second year of his residency he saw more, saw, actually, the precise diagnostic signs that would send alarm bells going off in a clinical setting. But she was not a patient and this was not a clinical setting, this was a warm bed with a hot, exciting woman—a woman who was, in addition, pregnant with his child.

Whenever he went over the story in his mind or in the telling, Alex felt as though he were reexperiencing arrows and knives that had pierced his flesh. As he articulated each detail in his memory he felt his skin tear, felt the warm blood run out, felt the cold burn of the blade's edge as it ripped through, as little tags of sensitive muscle and nerve were caught on the microscopic imperfections of the knife's edge and pulled off, screaming their messages to his brain.

This is what a parent feels. He remembered when Carmen was born, how he had cried at the sight of her, not for joy or sorrow or relief, but just at the sheer beauty of her. This living thing, squirming and crying, was of him in ways he could only sense, and was not of him, was of herself, in ways he could not imagine.

By the time Alex was director of his first clinic and a rising young star in the psychiatric circles of New York City, there was no

denying that his wife was schizophrenic. Her histrionics and paranoia were one thing, but then there was the New Year's Eve she
waded into the Central Park Reservoir and was pulled out babbling
about how she was looking for her lost womanhood, which her
husband had taken from her. The incident was kept out of the
papers. She was sent to a private clinic for several months. A nurse
was hired to take care of little Carmen during the day, but in the
evenings and on weekends, Alex took over her full-time care.

Alex was fascinated by his daughter. It was as though his nervous
system were in some miraculous way connected to hers. When she
was feverish and cranky he became excited, worried, and irritable.
When she fell or bumped herself he moaned and cried and soothed
her, trying to take the pain for himself. As it was with all her pains,
he breathed them into his own heart.

When she was hungry his body felt empty until she was fed. When
she learned to walk his own soul took flight.

Then Alex's wife came back from the clinic and life proceeded.
Of course, her illness was by no means cured or even under
control. Though there were always private clinics and opportunists
who claimed schizophrenia could be "cured," what the people who
knew better knew was that there was no such thing as a cure, that
whatever schizophrenia was did not go away. It might be controlled, it might lay dormant, its chaotic rhythms might in some way
be drugged or danced into syncopation with normal life—but the
discordant tones were always just a finger-fall away, the strings that
were tuned to another pitch pipe were always on the instrument.

So Alex found he was still responsible for Carmen's care most of
the time he was at home. Nurses were brought in, but Carmen's
mother fought with them, fired them, threatened them until they
quit. In the midst of this anguish, or despite it, Alex gave of his
substance to build solid pieces of his daughter's life. To support the
family and pay for the succession of nurses and private clinics, he
took on responsibilities he would have declined otherwise. He
bowed his head when he was proud or raised it when he was weary
because Carmen must be fed and clothed and kept warm and dry
and sent to school. Her little angers upset him more than even he
thought they should, but that was the way he was. When she smiled,
his life was a success.

Of course there were angers and resentments and passions. The child annoyed him, teased him, ignored him, interrupted him, refused him all sorts of courtesies. He yelled at her, spanked her, and felt guilt and self-disgust powerful enough to tame the barbarians. But his fierce love for her was not tamed. Once Carmen slipped from his grasp as they were getting out of the car and ran across the street into the path of a truck. The driver was alert and quick that day, and he stopped in time. But Alex's terror for his child ignited a fury within him and he swept her up with one hand and walloped her bottom with the other. Then he tugged at her outraged and rebellious little arm until she fell into a lockstep beside him, each of them burning with an inexplicable anguish, hating the other. But he hated himself more than she could ever hate him. He took refuge in being the parent, and explained his rage as righteous.

But Alex's pocket of little guilts became full and he emptied them into a sack that he carried on his back. He worked harder, bowed himself finally to his life, and gave more pieces of it to his daughter. With the ecstasy of a martyr he supported Carmen's fancies, solicited her girlish dreams. He did a pretty good job of it, too, he thought.

He looked back over his life and saw a messy, twisted trail of blunders, successes, passions, frustrations, guilts, and all the other detritus, both physical and emotional, we shed as we go on. But he felt that the pleasure he took in his daughter was so pure and so real that he could feel not only proud, but satisfied. All of what he thought was the meaningless jumble of his life might be coming to something. He might have been climbing to a place where the view was clear and far and good, after all. This was what life was about, he supposed. And that was fine.

Then, when Carmen was nine, Alex noticed the first sign. It was a balmy summer day, and father and daughter had gone down to the park to sail a toy boat. As the sailboat found the wind and heeled out into the lake, Carmen howled with glee. It was one of those moments when Alex felt so close to his daughter—just this simple act of setting a toy boat to sail in the pond and making the child laugh was more than enough. But, as if he had a sense of foreboding, he said to himself, "This is all I ask, this clear and beautiful moment." Carmen turned in joy to her father and the blue eyes of the daughter met the blue eyes of the father.

And then the child's face went blank and colorless. She shivered as if she were about to go into a convulsion.

"Daddy . . . I'm cold."

Alex put his arm around the girl, diagnostic checklists racing through his mind. Most likely a virus, he figured. But then the girl's eyes hardened into a gray stare. "It's Mommy . . . I want to go home. Mommy says I have to go home. It's too cold here."

Alex felt the ice spread out from his heart through his vitals to his skin. Now Carmen's shivering was intensifying and her eyes seemed to be rolling back into her head. The father snatched up his daughter, dropped the cord attached to the sailboat, and walked away.

But where to go? Alex thought for a brief instant, feeling his own foreboding increasing. He knew something unnaturally bad was going on and the idea of escape, of simply taking the girl to a private clinic to rule out a medical emergency . . . and then to the airport and disappearing in a faraway land. . . .

No, he was a physician and this was only his own foolish paranoia.

But when they got home, Carmen's mother was, indeed, in a rage. The broken vase and the forks and spoons on the floor in front of the television set told Alex that much. But when Carmen saw her mother come out from behind the living-room curtain, she struggled, made herself heavy, and dropped from Alex's arms and ran to her mother. Alex saw his wife's eyes turn black on him as the girl was lost in her embrace.

Alex was aware of the customs of primitive tribes toward those we call the mentally ill—the recognition at the first signs, the giving over to a shaman for special initiations. He tried that with his daughter, fashioning a contemporary version of such intensive analysis and care. He worked with the girl as a modern shaman might, testing her a little at a time, building her strength, trying with all the fierceness of his love and all the modern skills of his profession to untangle the already confused avenues of thought. Alex took the girl hundreds of miles away into the mountains for long weekends and tried to give her a deep, balanced keel of clear thinking so she might survive the stormy seas ahead.

But Alex's efforts were swamped by the inexorable progress of Carmen's deterioration, which was only intensified by the deterioration of her parents' marriage.

One day when Carmen was twelve she exploded at him. The explosion was lightning quick, and devastating. Alex was trying to make a decision about something she wanted, but his slow, methodical way of working through the options was irritating her. "How about if—" he started to say, but her arm waved across at him in a gesture of dismissal.

"Fuck you," she spat.

He slapped her face, backhanded, and could not speak for the rage that boiled up inside him.

He tried to make up a few hours later, but she unleashed a litany of fantastic accusations that left him speechless and numb.

The divorce took Carmen further away from him. The father-daughter trips to the mountains were labeled "eccentric, crazy rampages," and his wife, though just barely able to prevent herself from being institutionalized, was granted custody. The key witness turned out to be Carmen herself, who, according to Alex's attorney, went into the judge's chambers and, in response to the judge's questions, recounted a litany of Alex's sins against her and her mother—punctuated by a plea to the judge to please not let her father have her anymore.

There was nothing Alex could do. His visitation rights were sharply curtailed: He was not allowed to take Carmen outside the city limits, and he was not allowed more than four hours with the girl at a time, three times a month. Carmen was lost to him. There was an icy distance most of the time they were together. And when she wasn't defensive, when she opened up a bit and allowed Alex a glimpse of what agony was going on inside, the pain of watching his daughter's disintegration was too great for him. The visits dwindled.

They stayed in touch by telephone. There were more occasions when she could not be approached without her lashing out with sharp, cruel words and paranoid accusations. She would call Alex from college and ask for something. If the request could not be granted, or if he hesitated slightly while he tried to search for a way to help her, she would not wait, but would just bark "Fine," and hang up on him.

As a psychiatrist he was powerless. Carmen was not his patient, nor would she be anyone else's. As a father, he didn't know what to do. Every time he called her or drove down to have dinner with her he trembled inwardly for fear he might somehow provoke her venom. He was too vulnerable to it, he knew, but he could not tear himself away to a safe distance.

There were times when Carmen was as sweet and agreeable as she had ever been. But Alex grew to distrust these times. And so he felt himself farther away from her whether he liked it or not.

But the times when she was sweet and agreeable grew more and more infrequent. Alex stopped calling her, but she continued to call him and complain. Not about him, at least not at first, but about various things in her life. She was flunking out of college. She was losing this or that job. She felt too fat. Her insides were "all wrong." Then she would come around to blaming him, pointing out some early sin of his that could be shown to be at the heart of her current problem. She criticized him for both "ignoring" her and "dominating" her.

Sometimes she would whine at him. Other times she would calmly, almost obliquely, accuse him with a casual diffidence. She took for granted his responsibility for the disaster of her life. It was no big deal. Other times she would sic herself on him, releasing a torrent of vituperation. She would hang up before he could get a word in. He could tell when she was going to hang up because he would hear her screaming diminish in volume as the phone flew down from her face. Then it would crash and he would be left with an emptiness that even his own anguish couldn't fill. Their relationship was a war of attrition that lay waste to all of his sweet memories, even the memories of normal struggle and pain.

Alex stood farther and farther back from her. He found the distance painful, felt the hurt whenever he could not exercise his instinctive impulse to help her, whenever he hesitated for fear she might inflict some new outburst upon his vulnerability. He knew too well that his daughter had access to the most sensitive areas of his life, to the place where his connection with the universe was a living one—where he could see the reality of his own life in her life.

But painful as it was, Alex could not deflect the reflexes of his heart all the time. And there were times when his services were accepted without rancor or incident, when he actually was repaid with a smile or a quiet hour at her table with a glass of lukewarm fruit juice. But there was never a single moment they spent together when he didn't feel that both their lives were in some vitally significant way failures.

The thank-yous and the peaceful visits became rare jewels sparkling in the dim past, while the terrible outbursts and delusional recriminations grew not only more frequent, but more shrill. Though he knew the exact pages of the text where Carmen's symptoms and diagnosis were classified, in the depths of his anguish, where his knowledge and training deserted him, he felt she must be possessed. And as he weakened under the strain of fitting all of this into some picture of a loving, orderly universe—or even a scientifically limited one in which children did not become demonically possessed, but only ill—Carmen's life fell apart before his eyes. After many of her phone calls he wept for her and for himself.

When Carmen was hospitalized for the first time, Alex suddenly felt a warm gush of relief from the stone cold of his bitterness. At last, he thought, some order might be restored. *This is an illness, after all. My little girl is ill.*

His worst fears were that the seed that sprouted and bore fruit within his child was of his own sowing and that the genetic soup of his and his wife's making contained elements of old and new poisons that could not be eradicated until the entire potful was poured into the ground to mix back with the earth. There was no way of repairing her.

This was a fear the doctors sometimes tried to soothe but could not. The physicians could prescribe their drugs and make the voices and the paranoid delusions go away some of the time, occasionally even restore the mask of calm to her face. But this father always knew that deep in her heart his little girl felt a perfect, pure, and vicious rage, no matter how the pills obscured it in a pharmacological fog.

In Alex's case the reassurances were spoken and received mechanically, with almost-secret nods of acknowledgment and sympathy. Alex had delivered these same speeches countless times; he knew as well as the other psychiatrists that the words were more expressive of an attitude than a reality. Hope was a posture to lubricate with civility the friction between the professionals, who knew better, and the family, who knew how absurd and cruel and outrageous their lives had become.

When he was at his most philosophic and depressed Alex thought: Mine is only a single life, and hers one more. We are of no consequence. The stars will continue to burn whether or not we ever consume the life promised us in our dreams. And as his daughter periodically slid in and out between paranoid rage and a pale complacency with her medications and her stunted existence, he thought this: *I wonder if her heart burns as ferociously as mine with love for the life we can only imagine?*

Finally, Alex took advantage of a serendipitous job offer and spent the next ten years two thousand miles away from his daughter. The position at Bedloe State Hospital had brought him back to within a few hundred miles of his daughter's tormented life.

13

May was a dangerous month in the Bedloe Valley, a wanton lover who came with inviting arms and moist lips, kissing every infant bud. A warm promise was whispered on those kisses. *I will stay,* she smiled, *come out to me.*

Across the valley the ferns and grasses and leaves and flowers believed the promise and dressed the adolescent spring in shameless color. And while the competition among shades of pink and green and yellow flourished, the magnolia buds waited. A few peeled open just enough to send a tongue of white or purple into the sunlit air. Finally believing too, the magnolias shed their furry jackets and opened. The delirium of spring intensified as the heavy wet flowers pumped a liquorous scent out of their pink and purple centers. The earth danced day and night.

But brazen May was also a careless lover. In her breath there was icy treachery. One, two, three nights the frost came with cold teeth instead of soft lips, and each night bit harder.

The first morning the fruit flowers seemed stunned, but by the third morning they were shriveled. At least they left behind bright green leaves. The magnolias were not so graceful. Their gravid flowers, thick with syrup, began to rot on the branches. First they seemed to shrink, then brown veins spread over their fleshy petals. The more prudish buds survived, and within a few days there was enough life in the air and on the ground for the pastel celebration to continue. May was a lover who could not be denied.

Up the mountain, around Wendy's house, the cooler air had held back the flowers until after the last frost, so when they finally came, their blossoming was full and long. Wendy was kept busy for weeks picking flowers and colorful branches for bouquets, all of which she brought down to Wilson Cottage.

Wilson Cottage braced itself for spring. Greta Lampson was still depressed and suicidal. Her current antidepressant might as well have been a children's vitamin pill. Doc instructed all members of the staff to keep a close eye on her. In the evenings Zelda Glover lurked in the dark spaces of the unit and came out only to hand Wendy one small gift or another. One day it was a candy bar, another day it was a magazine she had bought at the hospital canteen. Wendy didn't realize how much she was letting her guard down until she was reading the magazine and came across a photograph in which the model's head had been neatly cut out of the page.

While Mary Johnson counted the comforts of an isolated corner of the Wilson Cottage dayroom, Henry Dove instructed three other male patients in the finer points of tuning a motorcycle engine. Henry's stock of motorcycle stories seemed to expand tremendously, and Dr. Rose was his favorite audience. Ethel Flynn, the newcomer who had shot her husband, asked Wendy if she could have a hair dryer to style her long hair. Wendy brought one in from home.

Most of the patients tried to get away with sleeping late, which Wendy, who had to wake them up when she arrived at work, attributed to spring fever. But on some mornings Wendy would arrive to find the entire unit just returned from a walk. The patients regularly cajoled the night staff into taking them to watch the dawn.

The tutelage of Steven Rose, M.D., continued. Under Doc's and Wendy's careful eyes he reviewed patients' medications and joined the fray in the treatment-team meetings, assisted Doc in therapy sessions, accompanied Doc and the unit psychologist in diagnostic and placement interviews, and observed various rehabilitation and nursing staff as they assisted patients with learning new skills. One of Rosey's favorite activities was to argue with Doc or Wendy over the use of certain psychiatric treatments, especially drugs, which he saw as "chemical straitjackets."

Rosey was a challenge, but the challenge wasn't to convince him of the ethical and medical rightness of psychiatry. Doc knew that defending psychiatry was a hopeless task as far as Steven Rose was concerned. What needed to happen was for Rosey to come to the same conclusion Doc had; that as a psychiatrist you tried your best with whatever tools you had at your disposal. And if you lived long enough or saw enough—or just plain wanted to help badly enough—you made the difficult decisions to use imperfect tools, including drugs that worked some of the time, didn't work other times, and did outright mischief a lot of the time.

But one of those drugs could probably take credit for saving Lily Speere's life, for having taken enough of the edge off her psychotic rage to lighten her hand as it pressed the glass into the flesh of her neck. She had drawn blood and made a scary mess in her bed, but she and Doc would have another chance.

"Look, Lily," Doc had said when he got back from his vacation and she was still in the infirmary recovering from her wounds, "I would like to work with you on your problems. But, you know, it's up to you. You almost put an end to it that night. And you can still do it. But you've got to make the decision. If you want to continue working, then fine. I'd like to. If you kill yourself, that's the end of it."

Lily had nodded and agreed not to kill herself.

It would be a race against time and whatever raging hurt within Lily's mind would drive her to lose all sense of proportion and self-worth again. The struggle was to build some middle ground. Because Lily's sense of self-worth had long ago been demolished—if it ever existed—Doc needed to create one.

Over the weeks he persevered and finally broke through Lily's resistance to taking responsibility for her life. This was a painful and courageous act for her, and he told her so: "I know how much it hurts, Lily, because yours is an imperfect life, a broken life. You'll always have your illness. Your strength and courage cannot change it, just as they didn't cause it. But you're one of the lucky ones, if you want to call it lucky. You have a fighting chance." A chance, Doc admitted, that depended upon her understanding that her thoughts and feelings were not always accurate reflections or responses to reality, but could be delusions generated from within her own mind.

Lily had nodded and freed a ribbon of tears to roll down her cheek. Doc made a mental note of that fact, with a string of mental gold and silver stars to mark its significance. Afterward, there was a subtle change in Lily, but one which Doc and Wendy noticed. Lily started helping Wendy with the flower arrangements, and sat next to her at meals.

[2]

An important part of Rosey's initiation into psychiatry was observing other units on tour with Doc. By April, he had toured the geriatric unit, the units for adolescents and preadolescents, and the Receiving Unit. Doc now figured Rosey was ready for the V-units, where violent patients lived.

We don't know what we are, or why, Doc believed. Scientists, theologians, artists, politicians all have their own ideas. A carload of psychiatrists will have a busload of opinions on the question. Doc wasn't sure himself, but, as he explained to Rosey while they were on their way to the wing of the hospital where the windows were heavily barred and the yard was ringed by a high mesh fence tipped with razor wire, he had found it safer and all around better medicine to assume that the same unfathomable energies found in one human skull were to be found in any other, regardless of the condition of the brain. He would concede that in each skull the vessels containing these furies and graces might be of different relative thickness, and when the brain was broken, they could be decanted in varying recipes for catastrophe. But the basic caldron of ingredients was the same for us all.

When they arrived at V-1, Rosey immediately noticed that the door was heavier than the door to Wilson Cottage. Not only was it locked tightly, but Rosey could see through the heavily wire-netted window on the door that there was a short hallway and then a second locked door. They had to ring for someone to let them in.

They heard the jangling of keys. The inner door opened and the tall, powerful figure of George Konopski, M.D., entered the hallway. He let the inner door close, but had the second door open in a few seconds. He held his arm out and used it to usher Doc and Rosey into the tiny chamber between the two doors. "I apologize for the sardine-can accommodations, but I want to make sure one door is always locked, that's all."

Doc looked at Rosey and nodded.

"Now stay behind me and . . ." Konopski's eye caught Doc's and sparkled. "Doc, you know the precautions in here. It's a lot of unnecessary bullshit most of the time. But every now and then, well, it sort of saves your life, and that's why you do it every time. Now just stay close to me."

Konopski opened the inner door and they were immediately in a medium-size dayroom, smaller than Wilson's. But then Rosey noticed that this ward had been partitioned. There was the usual nursing station strategically placed, with the usual glass walls from halfway up to the ceiling. But beyond the nursing station there was a second dayroom that was completely walled off with large, thick windows.

Rosey was instantly confused. There were about a dozen men standing around the first dayroom, and a few sitting on the sofas along the wall. Rosey picked out a man who was obviously a patient sitting on the sofa. The man was very thin, wore a tattered green T-shirt and jeans, and had shoulder-length, scraggly hair. He had both hands flat against his face and was rubbing his eyes, but there was an alertness about him that made Rosey feel uncomfortable: this man was not only aware of danger, he was capable of it.

There were two men in white T-shirts and dirty blue jeans leaning against a short stretch of bare wall across from the nursing station. They might as well have been standing on a street corner on a hot summer night. Their hair was crudely slicked back with water and they each had their thumbs hooked in their belt loops. Rosey felt their eyes on him.

Konopski seemed to move smoothly but quickly, his eyes open wide and constantly darting around the ward. Rosey caught a glimpse of a dumpy little man who seemed to appear out of nowhere off to their right side. Konopski held out his hand in a gesture that seemed defensive at first, palm out flat to deflect a possible blow, but actually became a friendly wave.

"Oh, hey there, Ned, howya doing, fella?" Konopski sang, like a politician, acknowledging the man, carefully appraising him and his relative value or danger, and then moving on. Ned, for his part, looked at the three physicians with wide, wet brown eyes, a child asking for approval or candy. "You're a good fella, Ned," Konopski waved again.

Rosey realized that Konopski had, of course, just passed by this man on his way to let him and Doc into the unit. Did he have to wave and reassure the man every time he passed him? Ned retreated to his chair and sat down.

Konopski stopped, his back to the glass wall of the nursing station. Doc took up position next to him. Rosey stood in front of him. "This is the V-unit 1," Konopski said. These men in here are all PCs, penal code patients. They've all committed extremely violent acts that the court system has decided were the result of mental illness. These guys are two-time losers. They've not only committed a serious crime and gotten caught, but they've been diagnosed as crazy, too. These poor bastards are getting both barrels from society!"

Rosey looked around. There were more men sitting on sofas in the dayroom behind him, men who seemed to blend in with the nondescript color of the wall. Only now they seemed to lean forward toward him. All except one, a short, blond-haired man who sat straight-backed, almost rigid, with his legs crossed. He wore a clean blue shirt and light green work pants. Must be a psych tech, Rosey figured. The man seemed alert, aware of everything in the room, but gave no sense of awareness of danger like the others.

"Excuse me, Dr. Rose," Konopski said to Rosey almost in a whisper. "One thing in here is don't turn your back on anyone, any of the patients, that is. Keep your back to the wall at all times." There was a note of cheery conspiracy in Konopski's voice. Doc chuckled as Rosey awkwardly looked around him and tried to position himself correctly. There was no way to be nonchalant about it.

"As I was saying, this is V-1, where the most violent patients are kept. V-2 is also for PCs and violent men, but the ones in there are not as violent. They're mostly sociopaths, con men. We've got a few of them in here, too, but mostly violent offenders here. Uhh, that's why the precautions."

A tall, burly, bearded man with a shaved head came out of the nursing station. He was wearing a leather vest and a chain bracelet. His light-blue jeans were torn at the hem to make room for his black cowboy boots. Rosey's eyes were drawn to the man's bare arms, which were littered with tattoos. The man smiled at Rosey and his gold canine gleamed.

"Oh, this is Frank Robbins, the meanest man who ever managed to get a job. Why, he's so mean, I'm surprised they let him out of the Navy. He's our acting nursing supervisor."

"He's . . . a nurse?" Rosey stammered.

Frank held out his hand to Rosey, who looked at Doc and then Konopski and then back at Robbins.

"For a man, he's all right," Konopski said sarcastically. "Of course, he lacks certain equipment that female nurses have that makes them more fun . . . but he can be a barrel of laughs in a short skirt and stockings. I don't blame you for not wanting to shake hands with him. I wouldn't if I were you."

Rosey had just started to extend his hand limply, drew it back, and then caught the joke and reached back out for Robbins's hand. Robbins seemed to bow slightly as he shook Rosey's hand. On second look, Rosey realized that although this was an incredibly strong man, his eyes gave away a gentle inner nature.

"Let's meet the rest of the crew," Konopski said as he led Rosey and Doc into the nursing station. Robbins noticed that Rosey was trying to walk and keep his back to the wall at the same time. He took up position behind the young doctor, who smiled gratefully.

There were two more men in the office, one sitting at the desk and the other standing in the corner. The man standing had long black hair and a dark, curly mustache. His eyes were sharp and smiling at Rosey. He, too, had several tattoos. The man who was sitting appeared less menacing, until Rosey noticed that his loose-fitting blue-green surgical blouse was hiding a massively muscled chest and arms like steel girders. Both men smiled easily.

"This rascal here is Simon," Konopski said, introducing the man who was sitting. "And watch out for this guy. Rocco, we call him, though the closest to Italy his family ever got was a bowl of spaghetti. His real name's one of those Wasp names that people tend to forget, so . . . what the hell was it, Rocco?"

Rosey realized he was in the middle of a private running gag. Rocco dismissed Konopski with a wave and shook Rosey's hand.

"Hey, Doctor Konopski," Rocco said with a leer, "heard the one about the Polish psychiatrist?"

Rosey was bewildered. The staff of this unit, as far as he was concerned, looked and acted like a motorcycle gang. And he was further confused when the skinny, long-haired man in the tattered green T-shirt approached the nursing station and walked right in, and kept coming toward him.

Rosey backed up a step.

"Oh, we almost forgot Jesse here," Konopski said.

Robbins slapped Jesse's back. "He's our undercover man!"

Rosey glanced around at all the faces and decided to risk shaking this man's hand.

"Glad to meet you, Doctor . . ."

Rosey realized he was waiting.

"Rose."

"Dr. Rose here is trying to make up his mind whether to be a psychiatrist or maybe go out and get an honest job," Konopski said.

Everyone in the room laughed, including Doc. Rosey allowed himself a weak smile. He was unaccustomed to the camaraderie of men like this, and he felt at a disadvantage.

"Well, Dr. Rose, now I'll tell you about some of our patients. We've got a celebrity or two here, you know." Konopski rested his hand on Rosey's shoulder.

"You met Ned there, Ned Salmon, the tough little guy that came up to us when we walked in. Ned's not a bad guy, really. I think he went sort of wild once and roughed up a bartender who was giving him a hard time. But I think he's okay. Wouldn't you say, Frank?"

Frank nodded solemnly. Rosey could tell that Konopski was very wise to include the other men in his evaluations. It gave them a sense of pride and participation. Robbins took the question seriously, as a consultation.

"Problem is, the state wants him out of here and he doesn't want to go. The public defender's suing for his release."

"What's the problem with that?"

"Well, Ned Salmon has been in here for six years. Before that he lived with his mother. She took care of him. But she's dead now. So he's going back to the streets. I don't think freedom is much of a gift for a man like him. He's scared all to hell and doesn't want to go."

"What's going to happen?" Rosey asked.

"They haven't set a court date yet. But we'll go in and tell the judge that we don't think he belongs out on the street, and the public defender will say we're restricting his civil rights and the judge will decide one way or the other. Probably let him go."

Konopski pointed at the glass-enclosed dayroom. "Over there is where we keep the real tough cases, the guys we really don't trust. We keep them over there because it gives us another barrier. See that guy over there, the boyish-looking one."

Rosey found the man, and he was boyish, except his eyes were tired and swollen and his reddish hair seemed dirty. The stubble on his face seemed to have a silver glint to it.

"His name's Dennis Kallikak. The way he tells it, his girlfriend begged him to smother her infant daughter, so he did. Then he says voices told him to strangle the girlfriend, so he did that, too."

"My God," Rosey sighed.

"Yeah, but wait a minute. He's not in here for hearing voices. My guess—and every other psychiatrist's guess—is that he didn't hear any voices at all. That's not why he got NGI and landed in here. No sir."

"Well, why then?"

"Well, when the police walked into the apartment, they found Dennis was still feeding the baby and, you know, having sex with the girlfriend—three days after he killed them. You've got to be pretty damn ill to do that, I think. Don't you?"

Rosey nodded, and swallowed hard. Kallikak had the same kind of blankness as all the patients in the room. A few sat stiffly as if they were strapped to their chairs. Then Rosey noticed that a few of the men actually were strapped in. Some of these men sat rigidly straining against the leather straps around their wrists, ankles, and waists. Others seemed to slump into the support of the straps. The room seemed cloudy, smoky, though no one was actually smoking. Most of the men sat on metal, straight-backed chairs. A few lumbered from one wall to the next. Two or three stood menacingly in the corner. Rosey recognized the dark stares. He had seen them on the faces of men standing on corners in front of bars or other hangouts. It was the look of the street, the unspecific glaring anger, the violence, restrained but always ready, the wide-eyed fear transformed into narrow slits of defiance and rage.

"Tell him about Tang," Robbins said.

Immediately the psych techs stirred and nodded. Konopski raised his eyebrows.

"Oh yeah, Tang, he's real interesting. See that little Asian guy strapped into the chair there?"

Rosey found the black shaggy hair and then the rest of the little shrunken man, almost lost in his clean white shirt. He stared straight ahead, apparently seeing nothing that was actually in the room.

"We just call him Tang. Nobody knows his name. Cambodian. Floridly psychotic. He was brought here by the police—came straight through, right to this unit, didn't even spend a minute in the Receiving Unit."

"Why?"

"I was getting to that. Our boy here went berserk at a professional wrestling exhibition down in the city. He climbed out of the audience into the ring and beat up all the wrestlers. You know those bouts are largely faked—"

"Yeah," Robbins interjected, "but those wrestlers are big mothers and they're excellent acrobats! And this little guy was throwing them out over the ropes."

"It seems our little fellow is a real expert in the martial arts. He makes the guys in the movies look like lame girl scouts, apparently. We've never seen him in action—and I hope to God we never do—but it took about twenty cops to get him down. Three of them landed in the hospital."

Robbins and the psych techs laughed.

"We'll keep him in those five-point restraints for awhile. Can't get too close to him without them. He's already kicked some staff and hurt them badly. We usually keep them on until we're sure the meds have taken hold."

"If they ever do," Robbins commented.

"Well," Konopski said, "I think they're working. He looks calmer today, doesn't he?"

Robbins looked at the psych techs, raised his eyebrows.

"Sure . . . . Doctor Konopski . . . when did you say you were going on vacation?" he said with a chuckle.

"You guys tear me up," Konopski laughed. "Anyway, we've sent his fingerprints to the FBI. If they've got anything on him, we should be able to at least find out who he is. Of course, that could take a few lifetimes. Unless the guy's suspected of being a communist spy, they take their time with this kind of stuff."

It was time to go. Doc rested his hand on Konopski's shoulder. "Well, George, I think it's time we got back to the real world of Wilson Cottage."

"Well, okay, Doc. If there's anything else I can do for you and Dr. Rose here, just drop by."

"Don't forget to get a look at our star patient on your way out" Robbins said as Rosey was shaking his hand.

"Oh?"

"Oh yeah, c'mon back in here for a minute," Konopski grasped Rosey's shoulder and gently but firmly pulled him back in the room. For the first time, the door was closed. "How could I forget our star patient?"

"Who?"

Konopski took on a conspiratorial air. "Don't point or stare, but you see that guy sitting all alone on the sofa in the dayroom?"

Rosey easily found the clean-cut man in the light-blue shirt. He had forgotten about him, though for a few moments he had wondered why the man had not entered the office, since he looked like a staff person.

"Well, does the name Linus Dillinger mean anything to you?"

Rosey thought about it, but did not remember the name.

"Think back about five, six years."

Rosey shook his head.

"Well, Doc, you remember, don't you?"

Doc nodded emphatically. "Oh yes. I sure do."

"Linus Dillinger kidnapped seven young women over the course of five months. He raped them, tortured them, and killed them. Blew their heads off with a shotgun. He was caught, convicted of seven counts of first-degree murder, and given the death penalty. While he was on death row, a woman journalist decided to write a series of magazine articles about him. She investigated his childhood, interviewed Linus himself, and did quite a job. The magazine articles became a TV movie—I can't believe you didn't see all this!

"Well, the upshot of it all was, Linus gets a new trial. She—this journalist—had made him famous. So now he's got the best legal muscle money can buy. And the verdict comes in same as before— guilty of first-degree murder. But this time they bring up all the stuff about his childhood and a lot of the crazy stuff Linus did on death row. And they get him sent here. He's not NGI. But as long as his legal muscle holds out and he's 'mentally disordered,' he's safe here. He can't be executed or sent back. He's officially a sick man. And brother, you better believe the state would like to send him back to death row. I'll tell you, there are a lot of high-priced egos involved here. State attorney general, governor, the works!"

Rosey looked at Dillinger, who sat calmly, securely—and looked up to return Rosey's stare. Their eyes met for a brief instant. Dillinger smiled, and Rosey looked away and blinked. He didn't see what Doc saw, which was the sad look that flashed through Konopski's eyes, the look of a man resigned to a struggle he didn't want.

14 _____

In the dark Wilson Cottage women's dormitory Greta Lampson lay on her bed and waited. The thin white sheet clung to her damp body like a gossamer shroud. She counted inside herself: *One. Two. Three. That's all of me. Just like Ingrid Bergman I am going to be.*

Everything was ready. There was only the waiting for the right time, for the silence to last long enough. Greta had heard Ethel Flynn get out of her bed and walk on light feet down the aisle between the beds. She knew it was Ethel from the sound her breathing made. And because ever since she'd come here that woman went to the bathroom at night more than anybody. Greta figured she'd dozed off and didn't hear Ethel come back.

[2]

Ethel had not come back. She had paused at the dormitory door just long enough to sense that no eyes would see her when she opened the door and slipped through the almost-darkness to where the bathrooms were. Ethel knew that there was a rhythm to the shadows. Maybe the wind blew the bushes and trees around outside and they made funny scary shapes that moved too fast on the walls and ceilings. Maybe the lights from passing cars made the shadows open like giant fans, and you could jump into it and move across the wall and then jump out as it shrank down to darkness. Maybe the shadows were alive, and if you made friends with them and danced your way through you would become one of them and no one would see you. Ethel knew this, and she knew how to dance with the shadows. No one had seen her dance across the room to the bathroom, had they?

As she slipped by she noticed that the night supervisor, a small Filipino woman, was sitting with her back to her watching a miniature television screen. That made shadows, too. There was someone else in the nursing station, another woman, asleep. Safely in the corner of the dayroom, undetected and at the threshold of the men's bathroom, Ethel thought the shadows were such loving partners.

Opening the door and getting in would disturb the shadows, Ethel knew, because the light was on in the bathroom. She could shut it off, but just opening the door would splash light into the dayroom. But there was a rhythm to this, too. She watched the flickering shadows on the wall and when they moved, she moved with them. The brief flash of light from the bathroom was lost amidst a crowd of other dancers.

As soon as she was in the room, Ethel found the light switch and welcomed the darkness. The room felt warmer, cozier in the dark. It didn't have to be a tile bathroom, it could be a hotel room with a fancy fountain right outside the window.

Ethel knew the bathroom was empty. She found her corner where she could watch the shadows and the door at the same time, and settled down into a crouch to wait.

[3]

Greta was done waiting. For her the waiting had been too long already. She counted in her mind: *One. Two. Three.*

One. She peeled off the sheet and rolled gracefully out of the bed into a crouch and then on to her hands and knees. She reached up under the mattress and found the papers and pulled them out, slowly so they wouldn't make any noise. One, two, three, four days of daily newspapers. Then she felt the springs up toward the head of the bed until she found the little box, the blessed little box.

Two. Greta sat back on the floor and let her back rest on the wall. She took a deep breath and tried to relax her pounding chest. She picked up one of the newspapers and began to slowly peel the pages apart. Ingrid Bergman was patient, that was one of her virtues. Greta assured herself she could be patient, too.

[4]

Ethel felt the quickening in her legs when one of the shadows turned out to be him, coming into the bathroom.

"Hey," he whispered with that gentle voice of his that Ethel loved.

"Here, honeyman," she whispered back from her shadow. She sat back and let her legs slip straight out in front of her. "I'm here."

"I can't see you."

Ethel could see that he was walking slowly with one hand stretched out in front of him, like a blind man or a sleepwalker. He was carrying something bulky tucked under the other arm.

"You brought your blanket. What a sweetie!" she said, in a voice that was almost too loud. "Keep coming, honeyman. I'm right down here. Mama's waiting."

He stumbled forward. "I can't see!"

"You don't eat your carrots. I watch you at dinner. You're a bad boy. You leave all your vegetables. That's why you can't see."

He laughed. He could see her now, sitting lazily in the corner. He took the last two steps slowly, then reached out for her hand.

Ethel slowly pulled him down to her. This was a dance, too.

"Roll out the blanket, honeyman," she cooed.

His mouth was hot and had a metallic flavor. Ethel closed her eyes and let him carry her down below the shadows.

[5]

Greta surveyed the mass of newspaper and crumpled clothes around her. In the moonlight it was a wasteland of rocks and black canyons. Now she pondered whether to lie across this land like a giant mountain goddess or stand piercing the sky and gather it up around her. *Ingrid Bergman knew how to die*, Greta thought. *She was a Swede, too.* Greta remembered the glorious thrill she got when she watched the smoke rising around the actress's face.

Greta made her decision. She got up, stood near the corner of the room beside her bed, and gathered the papers and clothes around her feet. They would not stay piled, however, and insisted on rolling down and spreading out. This would never do. She got an idea, and reached for the bedsheet. Because it was tucked in at the bottom, Greta had to tug at it until the mattress lifted and the sheet was released. Then she wrapped the sheet lengthwise around her shoulders into a loose, billowy gown. She had to bend over carefully in order to gather the newspapers and clothes under the gown. The top kept slipping, so she could arrange the newspapers with only one hand while holding the gown across her chest.

Three. Greta reached over and picked up the little box off the bed. She slid it open and carefully selected a single wooden match. The wood was colored gold. Greta had saved the matchbox from the day she found it in the visitor reception area. She knew she would use it someday.

The match lit in midstrike but the force of Greta's pushing it against the flint split it apart. She dropped it and got another one. This one she struck across the flint with a gentler stroke. It fizzled as she held it out in front of her—and then exploded into a bright, yellow-green flame.

Greta threw the box on the bed and bent over to light the paper under her gown. The green in the flame was gone now, turned all yellow-orange. And when the paper caught, and then the sheet, Greta's heart swelled as the first wisps of smoke sought and found her nostrils. Her eyes burned with a ferocious joy.

[6]

Ethel was not as careful on her way back to the dormitory. After all, wasn't it her right to get up to go to the bathroom, middle of the night or not? Of course, she had to be careful on the way to the bathroom. She could just walk right by the nursing station and say she was going to take a pee and who could stop her? But they would come looking for her when she didn't come back out in five minutes, even if they didn't see the man go in the same door.

But keeping her trysts a complete secret from the staff was a great game, and dancing with the shadows was too much fun.

The television was still crackling inane sounds of laughter, gun-fire, and clapping as Ethel slipped by across the dayroom to the dormitory door. She turned before opening the door, pausing with her hand on the knob to turn and dare the night staff to spot her. She found their silhouettes in the dark and let her eyes sparkle in the cheap white light of the television screen. She took a deep breath, smiled, and slipped quietly through the barely open door.

Ethel coughed at the sight of the fire. It wasn't the smoke, but the shock of the bright light where she expected more shadows. She tried to suck in more air to scream but her lungs were already full, and she gagged on the smoky air. For a moment she coughed and screamed at the same time.

Then she saw that there was a person in the flames, and she just yelled "HEY!" as loud as she could and started running toward the flames. She grabbed a blanket on her way down the aisle between the beds.

Her scream woke up several women, who immediately sat up in bed and screamed. Some just started to cry. But one of them, Lily Speere, jumped out of her bed and got to Greta before Ethel. She was pulling Greta off the pyre as Ethel arrived and started beating at the flames with the blanket. Ethel helped Lily lift Greta on the bed, where both women slapped out the flames.

"Get help! Get help! Get help!" Ethel screamed at the other women in the room, many of whom were now leaning toward the scene curiously. A few had gotten out of bed and were taking tentative steps closer to the corner. No one left the room.

Seeing this, Ethel started screaming as loud as she could. The fire was mostly out now and the room was as gray-dark as it had been before. But in the shadows she could see Greta's smoky face and Ethel pulled up a corner of the sheet and wiped at the woman's smoldering hair, stroking her gently as Lily's screams for help broke apart into sobs.

15 _____

There was something about Saturdays in May and June that made Doc want to get back to his office at the hospital and just relax, take stock, and perhaps do some unscheduled, gratuitous psycho-therapy. The show of spring colors was mostly over. The azaleas had bloomed late, but except for a few splashes of pink and purple here and there, the bushes had long gone to green, as had all of the flowering fruit trees. The rhododendrons had dropped the heavy petals of their flowers in the Memorial Day weekend rain. But in the first humid flush of real summer warmth after the rain, the honey-suckle had spilled their seductive scent and Doc couldn't take in enough deep breaths of it.

"I must have been a bumble bee in a previous life," he quipped whenever anyone caught him savoring the honeysuckle, walking right up and burying his nose in it.

There was honeysuckle right outside Doc's office window, so it was no wonder his Saturdays were always spoken for in June. More of his paperwork got done—though by no means all of it.

At the top of the pile on his desk, there were some sign-offs Wendy had left with a red balloon attached. That was her cute way of letting him know that this was paperwork that absolutely had to be done, otherwise he would have a stupid red balloon flubbing around his office with papers attached. Most of the sign-offs were medication records and changes that required Doc's approval. He had already discussed all of them with Wendy and the social worker. And even argued about some of them.

Lily Speere, for example, was doing well, making progress in her therapy, and Doc wanted to lower her dose of antidepressant. Wendy shook her head and said it wasn't a good idea, it was too soon. Doc fumed and fussed and had to wipe the sweat off his neck, but he also had to acknowledge, if only by a silent nod, that Wendy was probably right.

Ethel Flynn was doing well, if one considered being pregnant doing well. She seemed to think so.

Greta Lampson was not faring so well. Her burns had been too severe for the state hospital's infirmary, so Greta had been taken to Valley Municipal Hospital, which was a medical-surgical hospital with extremely limited psychiatric facilities. Now back in Bedloe's infirmary, her psychiatric condition was deteriorating even further. She refused to eat and had to be tube-fed. Doc had started the official bureaucratic procedure necessary to be permitted to treat her with electroconvulsive therapy, which he felt was her only chance. The question was, would the patient survive long enough for the court to decide whether she should get the treatment her doctor believed would save her life?

The papers signed, Doc took them, balloon and all, and placed them on Wendy's desk, which was so neat it made his look like the place where all the neat people threw their trash. But Wendy's desk was too neat, Doc thought. There was no photograph of a loved one to be seen, and Doc felt bad about that. He knew why there was no photograph, though Wendy had what you might call a loved one.

It wasn't any of his business, so Doc never spoke directly to Wendy about her affair with Bert, the male nurse from the other side of the hospital. But not speaking to Wendy about it didn't mean that he didn't think about it and shake his head inwardly—and outwardly when she wasn't looking.

Rosey had noticed Doc's shaking his head once as Wendy left the unit for one of her lunchtime trysts. "Are you concerned about her relationship with Bert?" Rose asked.

Doc did not want to talk to the young physician about Wendy, so he dismissed his inquiry with a wave. He could tell Rose was not baiting him, but that he really knew all about the affair, and most likely the source of his information had been Wendy, herself. That figured. Doc knew he was like a father to Wendy, which meant that he wasn't told about such matters. But Rosey was a friendly, non-threatening little-brother type. He would find out everything.

"It's none of my business," Doc had tried dismissing it again.

"She'll be okay," Rosey proclaimed. "She knows he's a jerk."

Doc had retreated into his office and shut the door.

[2]

There had been a time in Wendy's love affair with Bert when she forgot everything she knew, a time when all her mind could contain was Bert and her overwhelming feelings for him. That time had passed. She was drawn to him, but her knowledge of her own life was seeping back into her mind. And sometimes the knowledge was so acrid that Wendy marveled at how she ever could have put it aside, even for love.

But that was part of a woman's life, after all, wasn't it, she asked herself over and over again, to love and suffer and forget? Wendy knew this not from her own experience so much as from the stories of other women. Especially Nelly, a nurse supervisor who had worked at the hospital when Wendy had first started, years ago. Nelly had taken Wendy as her favorite, perhaps because she had seen the way Wendy's face opened up in pure admiration and awe whenever the two were together. Wendy saw in the older woman all that she wanted to be: a strong, sure, able professional who was tough but compassionate. And sexy. Wendy saw the way the men looked at Nelly—both the staff and the patients.

Wendy's first assignment at Bedloe had been in one of the V-units, V-2. The men in V-2 were mostly PCs, but, unlike the men in V-1, their crimes had not been as violent. The ward was populated by psychopaths of varying degrees of competency. Wendy, at first, believed that a psychopath was necessarily "an axe murderer or something gruesome like that." Nelly explained to her that psychopaths were not necessarily killers at all, but just people who were "a little deficient in the conscience department, that's all. Most of them are just con artists." Nelly assured her, "You can handle them just fine once you know that they're always up to something."

And handle them Nelly did. She took no conning or intimidation from anybody, whether it was a patient or a physician.

Then one day she disappeared. She didn't show up for her shift, and calls to her home received a "disconnected" recording. The staff was mystified.

Two days later, one of the patients of V-2 disappeared, Robin Stokes, a young, wiry, handsome fellow who had been admitted to Bedloe after committing a series of bizarre kidnappings. Robin would kidnap someone and then hold them for ransom. But the victim was usually a housewife or a single mother. Robin never bothered the women sexually. He seduced them to the point where they sort of trusted him—a task for which he had an uncanny knack—and then tied them up and drove off with them. Then he called their homes and demanded unrealistically large ransoms. For the "safe, unharmed return" of a thirty-eight-year-old mother of four who lived in a mobile home, Robin demanded of the husband a ransom of $250,000.

All of the kidnappings ended with police SWAT teams and hostage negotiators surrounding Robin's hideout. There would be a few tense hours until Robin would let them know that he was unarmed. There would be some tear gas, some storming of the hideout, and then Robin would be brought out in handcuffs. There would be a trial, at which Robin would be found not guilty by reason of insanity and sent to the local community mental hospital. Within a few months he would escape or be released and move to another state. Since he had committed the last three kidnappings in the same state, he had been sent to Bedloe "for a good long stretch."

Nelly and Robin were apprehended by the state police about two hundred miles from Bedloe. At her hearing, Nelly professed a passion for "this poor victimized man" that brought tears to the eyes of most of the people in the courtroom, including the judge.

Since she had not actually helped Robin escape from the hospital, charges against her were dismissed.

But so was she, from her job at Bedloe.

Wendy was shaken. All she could think of was all the times she and Nelly used to talk about "those women," referring to the wives and girlfriends of the PCs at Bedloe. At least half of the PCs in V-2, and about one-third of the men in V-1, had wives or girlfriends who not only visited regularly, but actually followed them as they were moved back and forth between the state prison and the state hospital, as either their mental states or their favor with the administration changed. Wendy and Nelly would see them and talk to them when they came in with what Nelly called "the attempts at baked goods" for their men. "My God," she would say to Wendy when the visitor was out of earshot. "I can't understand it, Wendy. If you want to save somebody, join the Peace Corps or something. If you want to kill yourself, jump off a bridge—it's quicker."

Wendy would nod silently.

Wendy went to see Nelly after the hearing. It was an awkward meeting. Neither talked about the hospital or the hearing or really anything of substance. Wendy talked about her flower garden. Nelly talked about moving to another state and "trying something new," as if it was a daring career move she had been dying to make all her life, a real lunge for freedom.

Then, as Wendy started to leave, perhaps Nelly could see the ashen vacancy on the younger woman's face, which came not only from disappointment and confusion but also from embarrassment. She also saw that there were questions Wendy wanted to ask, but couldn't. And even if she could, Nelly could never answer them. So, just before Wendy got up, leaving her iced tea untouched, Nelly smiled bitterly and looked away, out the window at the wind skewing the snowball bush, and said, "Shit. He wasn't worth a fart and a half in bed. I should've known."

Not long after that, Wendy became involved with Bert. She knew going in that he had a reputation and that he wasn't "what I want in a permanent relationship." But none of the things she knew stopped her, for passion can neither be stopped nor started by things known. Wendy felt a ferocious appetite to devour and be devoured by this man. Even if—or perhaps because—he gave of himself in the most niggardly, constipated, teasing fashion, Wendy could see in the sparkle of his shadowy eyes a depth of wanting that promised heaven. It wasn't until just recently that she had begun to suspect that the desire was her own reflected back, and the promise was the neglected spirit of her own lust.

But she went to him, still, thinking maybe that's all you can expect in life is to see your own love reflected in a pair of pretty eyes. "After all," Wendy excused herself, "I'm young and there's plenty of time for fun and business." It was a good way of denying her own frustration. She settled for a crumb and believed that it was somehow connected to the cake, denying that if it were in any way connected to the cake it would not be a crumb, would not feel, or taste, or fail to satisfy like a crumb.

She went to him and in their hot secret tugging and thrusting denied and forgot and, when she came out empty, learned all over again.

"Oh, Wendy," he said with that infuriating smile as he lay back on the sofa and rested his hands under his head and looked like he had just eaten the world.

Wendy tried to wipe the sulk off her face, but when she turned to smile at him in what she thought was a "satisfied womanly way" it was still there and she knew it. She saw him look at her and glance away.

Wendy's smile vanished.

Bert inspected her. Wendy could tell he was trying to make a decision.

"If you're unhappy, we can stop doing this," he said calmly.

Wendy just talked now. "No, I don't want to stop. I just . . . I . . . I just want to leave, that's all. My lunchtime's almost over. I'm nervous about being missed."

They both knew that she was hardly ever nervous about being missed. This was her break time, and as for the possibility of being discovered, that was not a consideration. This stretch of hall happened to be the longest possible route between two parts of the hospital that didn't support a lot of back and forth traffic in the first place. There were no occupied offices, so it was a forgotten place.

He gave up, finally, "Yeah . . . okay. I'll see you, lover, okay?"

Wendy nodded, smoothed out her slacks and left. He had won again, she realized. She wasn't ready to not come back to this place, not ready to face the dissolution of all her fantasies. Not ready to find out that he really needed her, and, worse because with it came heavy responsibilities, that she didn't need him.

But she felt how strong and supple her thighs felt as she walked back to the unit. Her whole body tingled, and this made her feel proud. She was still young, after all.

16

[1]

The blunt realities of mental illness shatter our most deeply held convictions about the nature of human consciousness and behavior. Diseases that attack the brain appear to possess the soul of what makes us moral, responsible, even spiritual human beings. The mentally ill are more different from us than we imagine and more like us than we care to admit. They have crossed a line that separates them from us biologically, behaviorally, and sociologically. We may cross that line, too. Though our science and our religion and our laws try to tell us where that line is and what we must do to stay on the safe side of it, advice and rules are the flimsy constructs of fear. Mental illness makes a cheap mockery of all of it, and then shatters it. Mental illness turns all wisdom into lunacy.

Mental illness is not a matter of will or moral strength. Just as there is a difference between a broken arm and a healthy arm, there is a difference between a broken mind and a healthy one. A broken

131

arm may not lift or guide or hug or hold, or it may falter or feel unbearable pain when it tries. So will a broken mind.

We want to believe the mind is inviolate and independent from physical infirmities, and that a mentally ill person is, for whatever reason, separated from it, *out* of it. That is not the case. The mind is only the brain in action. The mind is a fiction, a brilliant fantasy created by the brain to fool itself, to elevate its importance and hide its physical nature, to hide the fact that it can break in more places than an arm, and that when it breaks, there is no safe but hidden chamber of reason that we need only to find and reenter.

When the mind breaks, all sinews and muscles of behavior may be broken, from the innermost sensations of consciousness to the outermost manifestations. A broken mind may drift in a storm of stimulation from inside and out, or it may languish, a stone on a dead shore. A broken mind may see what is not there and fail to see what is. It may feel hate when love is called for, joy at others' pain, or unbearable torment from a child's laughter.

All thoughts and sensations, all passions, all desires and fears and appetites, all memories must trudge across the miscreated landscape of the broken mind. What they bring home from this journey may be a bag of fragments, crumbs of love and shards of rage.

But though the brain may fool itself with its invention of the mind, this is minor mischief. The brain does not break itself, it does not choose illness or stumble into it because of a misread map of life. The mind is not lost because a weak brain drops it along the way. The madness of the mentally ill is not a matter of will or strength or guidance.

But neither is our sanity. The mentally ill may have crossed a line, but our lives weave along the same delicate borders. We are not so different from Walter Channing or Lily Speere or Carmen Greco or any of them. We wonder what comedies and tragedies are waiting for us upon our life's journey, but we forget that the threads of our magic carpet's tapestry of consciousness were dyed in the same mammoth gene soup as theirs. Our civilized ideas and decisions and dreams are stretched taut on the same loom, and cut with the same clumsy shears.

Nowhere is the cutting more savagely ragged than in schizophrenia, where, despite popular romantic notions, the mind is not neatly split, but left in shreds.

You'll hear it on radio and see it on television, you'll read it in magazines and newspapers and even books, your friends will say it: *I feel so schizophrenic today. Half of me wants this and half of me wants that.*

Or: *She's a real schizo. Sometimes she likes me and sometimes she hates my guts.*

Or: *He has a schizophrenic personality. A real split personality.*

You will not hear it in the home of Fran Channing or other members of the Family Organization. You will not hear it in the offices and wards of Bedloe State Hospital.

For if schizophrenia is splitting, it is not the fine cleaving of the mind into neat halves, it is the kind of splitting a sledgehammer performs on a crystal chandelier, the kind of splitting a freight train visits upon a wedding cake. Schizophrenia splits the mind like a rock splits a flower. Schizophrenia is smashing, not splitting. It is not an argument between friends of different dispositions, but a cacophony of feuding relatives, angry children, and mortal enemies playing musical chairs with their roles. It is not a team on a bad day, but a stadium of strangers who have forgotten why they are there.

Schizophrenic people do not have trouble deciding between love and hate, good and evil, right and wrong, east and west, pizza and Chinese. Rather, their inner lives are a World War III of tension, combat, and attrition. Every menu they look at has them on it.

It is not enough to say that a schizophrenic person has hallucinations and delusions, that he or she hears or sees or suspects what is not there. It is barely enough to say that the schizophrenic lives in a consummately magical universe, where everything is up for grabs. Laws of physics, chemistry, biology, astrology, gravity, economics, the federal government, the Geneva Convention, the jungle—do not hold fast, they square dance on thin ice.

Think you know all about this so-called splitting?

Bring the symphony orchestra onto the gridiron and hand them footballs. Bring the football team into the auditorium and hand them the instruments and sheet music. Try driving on the wrong side of the road, convinced you're right. Try passing a multiple-choice test written not in ink but in live fleas. Try feeling the next moments of the life of the world depend on whether or not you blink your eyes.

Alex Greco learned this in school, but the real lessons were delivered by his daughter. Fran Channing, too, learned about the borders crossed by the schizophrenic. She spoke to Walter regularly. As long as he was able to keep her telephone number straight, he could call her on a public phone made available to patients.

Each call was a lesson. The humming and screeching and obscenities ebbed and flowed around Walter's stammering voice. Walter reported on the goings-on in the unit from his own perspective. Fran knew Walter's thinking could be disorganized, paranoid, or delusional, but she also knew the horrors of D-7 firsthand. She was always surprised at how well he bore up. On his bad days he complained and shared with Fran some of his delusions about how his body parts were being electronically surveyed by the CIA and the Korean government, of which Dean Lester, M.D., Penny Scott, and most of the staff of D-7 were agents. On his better days he complained and rattled off a long list of offenses against him by staff and other patients. More often than not he just vaguely referred to these incidents as if they didn't bother him and tried to reassure his mother that he was all right. "I'm fine, Mama," he would say in a way that sounded to Fran like someone had taken the melody and rhythm and timbre of his voice, shattered them, and then stuck the pieces back together with cheap glue, "Don't worry, because I'm fine, I'm fine, I'm fine."

March had been a relatively good month for Walter, owing, perhaps, to his time in the Bedloe infirmary. Soon after he returned to D-7, Dean Lester thought it might be a good idea to change Walter's medication, because, after all, there had been some trouble with this patient and he knew the record could be closely examined in the future. To change a patient's medication, he had to have the approval of Walter's treatment team.

A treatment team consists of all the members of a unit's staff who have responsibilities for a patient's care. The usual team will have a psychiatrist, a psychologist, a social worker, one or more psych techs, a registered nurse, a rehabilitation therapist, and perhaps other special therapists or hospital staff who might work with the patient. At a treatment-team meeting the members gather to discuss a patient's condition, progress, and needs. Are the medications working? Does the patient need a higher dose? A lower dose? A different drug? What has been going on that everyone responsible for this patient should know about? Any assaults on or by the patient? What's the patient been talking about in therapy and around the unit? In theory these issues, and more, would be passed around, examined, argued over—and decisions would be made and noted on the patient's record.

Very little went according to theory in D-7. Whereas treatment-team meetings in other units could be the scene of passionate disagreements over the best course of action for a patient's care, no one ever argued in D-7, unless it was over adding a new responsibility to the staff's roster. Whereas the meetings in other units often went overtime and had to be extended because there was so much to cover, the D-7 meetings covered every patient in a single meeting and usually broke up early.

And whereas staff in other units could be cajoled into discussing treatment-team meetings with relatives of patients, in D-7 such requests were flatly denied or ignored. In the days immediately before and after the meetings, phone requests to speak with staff members, most of them long distance, were put on hold and left to languish for minutes before being "lost in transfer." If, by chance, a message was taken, the call was not returned.

The discussion of Walter's medication change in the D-7 treatment-team meeting consisted of mechanical nods and a general request for a cigarette by Penny Scott.

Fran noticed a change in Walter during his first call in April. His agitation seemed closer to the surface and he neither complained about the unit nor tried to comfort her. Claiming that he had "new knowledge about the incidents," he accused her of beating his dog Scruffy while he was in school. Fran tried to field these statements calmly. But if she tried just letting them go by, Walter seemed to grow angrier. If she disputed his claims, he simply repeated them and said he knew and she didn't have to hide it from him anymore. After half an hour, Fran wrestled the call to where she and Walter agreed to disagree on the facts and she ended the conversation. That night she called the D-7 nursing station seven times and was put on hold and eventually disconnected every time. She called the hospital switchboard and was merely put through to the unit again. And then disconnected.

Finally, Fran made the call through an operator, instructing the operator that it was an emergency call and that she had to speak to a responsible person in that unit. The operator responded to the urgency in Fran's voice, and the night-shift psych tech responded to the presence of a witness on the line. There was no psychiatrist on duty in D-7 that night, so one was hustled out of another unit. He found Walter's chart and told Fran that her son's medications had been changed several days earlier.

Fran called D-7 first thing in the morning. She did not waste any long-distance calls because she used an emergency operator first time around. She demanded to speak to Dr. Lester. The psychiatrist calmly explained that they were trying "something new" with Walter and that "some early adjustment difficulties" were to be expected. He ended the call by reassuring her and telling her to "call anytime."

[2]

Dr. Steven Rose had not had the benefit of such long-term schooling as Fran had received. He had completed most of the assigned reading in medical school and had attended lectures in which schizophrenia was discussed on one day as if it were a psychobiological catastrophe and on another day as if it were a spiritual opportunity, a blessing dressed by an evil culture in the cloak of a curse.

Doc decided it was time for Rosey to visit D-7.

On the way over Doc gave a little introduction to the unit. "D-7 is one of the 'back wards' of the hospital, one of the places people talk about when they talk about how awful a state mental hospital can be. It's the ward where the most chronic, most seriously ill patients are kept." Doc paused and contemplated for a moment on the word he had used. "That's an interesting word, 'kept,' " he said. "I guess in this case it fills the bill, because that's about all that's done with many of these people. They're 'kept.' These are the toughest cases." Rosey was silent.

"You'll see."

When they first walked in, Rosey decided nothing could have prepared him for D-7.

They were immediately engulfed in the buzzing action of the

twin dayrooms. Men flittered by. Men paced, frittered nervously with their hands. There was an unintelligible shout from an unseen corner of the room. Rosey was knocked back by a humid wave of fetid odor. All of a sudden he felt damp and somehow stained all over and inside his clothes, as if the filth sought out the surface of his body and stuck to it. All Rosey could think about was a barnyard, and flies, and oppressive heat.

"Fuck you!" a small, grizzled patient shouted at another man who was walking away from him. The grizzled man swatted at the other man, but he was too far away to hit.

There was a scream from the corner of the room. Rosey turned and saw a tall, thin man standing over a short, fat, and much younger man. And the thin man was clutching the younger man's shoulders and shaking them, all the time beaming a demonic, toothless grin. The younger man was terrified.

"He's hurting that man," Rosey said.

Doc nodded. He looked around and saw no staff, so he took a step toward the corner.

The young man screamed again. The thin man saw Doc take the step, his eyes were caught in Doc's for a wild second, and he immediately looked away and released his grip on the younger man's shoulders.

There was too much to keep track of. "Get outta here!" a man cried, just a few feet from Rosey. The young physician cringed, and turned toward the cry, expecting a blow. But he saw that a man dressed only in pajama bottoms was slapping at another man who was pulling on his pants leg.

"Hey," Rosey said. "Leave him alone."

The two men looked at Rosey as if they had just become aware that he was in the room. Both seemed to shrink as their eyes went blank and they looked away. The one who had cried at the other made one final swipe with his hand and walked quickly away.

Rosey felt dozens of eyes on him now and was uncomfortable. He tried to hide from the eyes, from the wide, ominously vacant stares of the men, but found that he could not. Though empty, the stares were far from neutral. The men's eyes were like stillbirths. There was a lifeless, tragic pregnancy to them. They carried death, wished for it, or poured it out. Rosey shuddered.

All of a sudden he realized Doc was walking quickly away and was not aware that he was leaving him behind. Doc was striding across the room, making his way through the crush of men toward the nursing station between the two dayrooms. Rosey whimpered an unintelligible syllable and hurried to catch up with him.

Doc stopped at the nursing station and, when he saw that there were two people sitting in the room, seemed to compose himself.

"Is Dr. Lester about?"

Penny Scott casually dragged on her cigarette and looked up at Doc. She shook her head.

"I see," Doc murmured. "Well, I'm Dr. Rush. I'm giving my resident, Dr. Rose, a tour of the hospital and I arranged with Dr. Lester to show him this unit today." Doc looked at his watch. "We've got another appointment, so I'm going to get this over with now, if that's all right with you."

Penny Scott looked away from Doc, glanced at the other woman in the room, then shuffled some papers on the desk. She took another slow drag on her cigarette then shook her head irritably. "They never tell me about this stuff," she spat. "And I'm supposed to be the supervisor. Hell I am!" She shook her head with a bitter kind of petulance and without looking at Doc just waved him through. "Go ahead."

"Thank you," Doc answered with an almost jovial politeness.

Doc took Rosey by the arm. "Let's take a look around," and he led him away from the nursing station.

"Aren't you going to tell that woman about what's going on?" Rosey insisted.

Doc tugged at him. "Sure. Come with me. Into the dormitory."

Rosey looked back at the woman, as if he might say something to her, but when he saw her staring at him with an intensity of scorn and suspicion that he had never before felt directed at him, he gave up his resistance to Doc's tugging and followed him.

"Hey you! Hey you! Hey you!" a naked man in their path machine-gunned at them.

As soon as they were in the dormitory, Doc took a quick look around and then pulled Rosey into the corner. He did it gently, as if that was the exact right place for them to go all the time, and had nothing to do with Doc's wanting to pass on any secrets.

Doc turned to Rosey, but he saw that the young man's attention had been drawn away into the room, to a man sitting on his bed masturbating. Across the aisle there was a man lying on the floor, wrapped in sheets pulled down off the bed. He looked as if he were a big fish that had been netted in the sheets.

Rosey squeezed his nose at the acrid smell of urine in the room.

"I didn't want to say anything where that hag could read my lips," Doc said. "She does that, you know. And the legend is that she has eyes in the back of her head to do it, too."

"This ward is a disgrace!" was all Rosey could say in response.

"No," Doc shook his head. "It would take a lot of work to get it that good. A disgrace is when you've got too many patients and they're not getting as much care as they should. A disgrace is what most of the hospital is—in fact, is what most of our entire mental health system is, on a good day. This ward is a lot worse than that."

Rosey couldn't restrain his own bitter, amazed smile—for there was the wry, curious curvature of Doc's mouth that seemed to say, *Whatever horrors my eyes see, I'm entertained by it.* Doc seemed to be observing life from a different perspective.

"Why doesn't somebody do something about it?" Rosey finally asked.

"Young man, are you asking that question as a philosopher or as a politician?"

"I'm asking as a physician."

"This ward has a physician."

"Well, where is he?"

Doc raised his eyebrows and shook his head. "This is a problem ward. Nobody denies that. These things aren't easy to fix up."

"Well, I—"

Rosey's plea was interrupted by a moan from the other side of the room. Both doctors turned . . . and saw that it had come from underneath a rumpled pile of sheets on a bed in the far corner of the room. As they hurried over, the moan came again, louder.

"Maaaamaaaa, I hurt!" The sick pile of sheets stirred. There was a spasm and two feet jerked out straight at the end of the bed. Doc got to him first and his trained eyes went first to the young man's head, which was red and ripe with moisture. Little droplets of sweat born from the anguish of his flesh merged into rivulets that trickled down and soaked the sheets. Rosey could feel the heat from two feet away.

"He's burning with fever!" Rosey exclaimed.

"Hmmm." Doc murmured.

Suddenly the young man spasmed again and his hands convulsed as if they were wings and he was trying to fly away.

"Ohhh Maamaaaa maamaa mama mamaaaa!" the young man cried.

Doc reached down and touched the young man's abdomen. He shook his head.

"What is it?" Rosey asked.

"Don't know. Could be pneumonia. Could be worse," Doc said. Doc turned and politely, but firmly, pushed Rosey out of his way as he left the bedside. "Let's go."

Rosey stood firm. "Let's go! What do you mean?"

Doc kept going. "We've got to get this boy to a hospital."

Rosey half-laughed, half-cried. "This is a hospital! And we are doctors!"

But Doc had not waited. He was out of the room. In a flash he was in the nursing station. Without waiting for polite formalities, he ignored the two women and picked up the phone and quickly punched the number.

"That's an outside line, it better not be long distance," Penny Scott said with lazy bitterness.

Doc ignored her, in fact, his eyes didn't even see her, though they were aimed right at her.

"Emergency dispatcher. We need an ambulance at Bedloe State Hospital. Immediately. We have a young man here with a severe systemic infection."

Doc took a deep breath.

"No, he's not at our infirmary. He's in D-7. I'll have our security car meet you at the gate to get you here."

Doc took another deep breath as he listened to the question. "No, I don't know the patient's name."

For the first time Doc looked at Penny Scott and saw her, saw that she was watching him with her eyes narrow, fearful, and mean. That's all he saw.

"No," Doc said. "Nobody here knows his name."

17 _____

[1]

The toughest thing Alex had to do in May, tougher even than fielding three distraught, barely coherent phone calls from his daughter Carmen, was calling up Fran Channing to tell her that her son Walter had almost died from pneumonia. The woman had started to cry, almost choked on her sobs, then apologized because she felt embarrassed. Alex assured her that Walter was out of danger and resting comfortably at Valley Municipal Hospital. Fran thanked him for the information and then excused herself to call the other hospital.

Alex felt trapped inside Bedloe. The many administrative skirmishes with Sam Akbar wore him down. A hospital existed, as far as Alex was concerned, to perform medical procedures to help the sick. In the case of the mentally ill, when healing was not possible, help translated into asylum. If the hospital could not remove the illness, at least it could provide an environment where the patient suffered the least. Alex knew that this was all that could be expected for most of Bedloe's patients. The trouble was that Sam Akbar had another philosophy: the hospital existed as a cog in the bureaucratic machine, a workshop for Sam's ambition. From day to day, Sam's goal was to keep the hospital running smoothly. If that meant ignoring medical obligations, bullying staff, and allowing the detritus of neglect to accumulate and fester, well . . . as long as certain numbers made a satisfying sound when crunched in the state government's teeth, all was well.

The latest skirmishes, as usual, were over the medical staff's desire to improve the quality of care. That Sam was unresponsive to the medical staff was a given at Bedloe. When, at Alex's urging, the psychiatrists had formed a committee to investigate, monitor, and improve laboratory and clinical procedures, Sam ignored them. When they made recommendations, he refused to recognize them as a valid administrative body. "Who are these people?" he barked at Alex. It was one of a long series of battles, and looming over it was Alex's knowledge that he could press too vigorously, lose his knack for administrative diplomacy in the face of Sam's unique crudity, and provoke his own dismissal.

When Alex considered the likely trashing of his career and it didn't seem all that unpleasant a prospect, he knew it was time to get away. Besides, Alex was subject to the same restlessness spring engendered in everyone else. Fortunately, his professional organization, perhaps because it was composed of people who made a life's work out of the human mind and its zigzag course, had the foresight to schedule its national convention on the cusp between May and June.

Alex had made his plans months before. He knew that by going away from the hospital, by taking his professional eye elsewhere, his focus would be clearer when he returned. Bedloe State Hospital, after all, existed in a bigger world, and Alex needed to have that awareness reinforced. He always found his dedication strangely reinvigorated after he stepped back and viewed psychiatry and the care of the mentally ill as depicted in the quick, long brushstrokes of the convention.

Alex thought he would someday do a painting of the convention. It would be a picture of a carnival. Not a church carnival, although the convention had its patron saints. Not an ethnic street carnival, because the food wasn't that good. No, the national psychiatric convention was a combination trade show and state fair, with its midway barkers, its bizarre exhibits of the horrors of nature and man, its jerry-rigged rides, and its blue-ribbon barnyard. Despite the protests of his serious nature, Alex looked forward to it.

The gaiety seemed natural. At the convention mental illness and its attendant problems and tragedies were matters to be discussed in workshops and classes. Drugs were not a matter of life and death, sanity or psychosis, but products to be marketed. Here, the battle against madness could be contained in slogans, pamphlets, advertisements, symposiums, speeches, and films. The battle was at a safe distance for a few days, more like intellectual wrestling than hand-to-hand combat. By the end of the week, all would be back at the front.

The anthill grandeur of the scene never failed to both amuse and fascinate Alex. Dozens of buses pressed into service as shuttles converged on the front of the convention center, which looked like a vast aircraft hangar rising out of the concrete bunker around it. The red, blue, green, and yellow buses were the only splashes of color against the bone-white of the center. The people emerging from the buses were uniformly gray, brown, and black forms spilling out in a compact line, spreading out on the terrace, and then clotting into crowds to get through the few doors that were open.

Alex's bus slowly made its way through a crowd of demonstrators who were blocking the driveway despite the best efforts of the police. They parted, but very slowly, to allow the bus to inch forward. As the bus passed, they pressed their signs up at the windows. *Psychiatry Kills*, Alex read. The demonstrators' faces had a blank, almost affectless anger. Alex examined their eyes and found the stone rage of righteousness.

Alex got out of his bus and immediately his eyes were drawn to a circle of about a dozen men standing around one ragged man with shaggy long black hair and a beard who was sitting on the sidewalk. Walking by slowly, Alex overheard the curbside consultation.

"I was in there for three months and all they did was fill me up with drugs. They wanted to zap me with their electrodes but my lawyer wouldn't let them," the ragged man said.

"What medication were you on?" one of the psychiatrists asked him. The others nodded.

"Hell, man, vitamin H."

Several of the psychiatrists nodded.

"Are you getting any care at all?" another psychiatrist asked.

"Yeah, I stop in every now and then."

"Are you having any hallucinations?"

"I don't have time for hallucinations, man. It takes all my energy to keep ahead of the FBI."

Alex walked on toward the crowds funneling into the black-glass face of the convention hall.

Inside, the hall seemed to open up in much larger proportions than seemed possible from its outer dimensions. As the floor spread away, the ceiling rose twenty, thirty, forty feet or more in a maze of glass. Alex had to step outside the stream of people for a moment and stand still to gain firm footing as the swarm of psychiatrists spread out toward different destinations. Some hurried for the stairs and escalators. Some took their places in line at the appropriate registration desks. Some just seemed to be headed toward no particular point, though they appeared quite purposeful.

After registering, Alex headed down the escalator to the exhibit floor, which was a football-field-size room arranged into more than a dozen aisles of booths. As he descended, the panorama of the exhibit hall spread out below him. The middle aisles were dominated by several large islands. There were three huge garden tents, all in bright shades of green, pink, blue, and yellow. There was a minitheater constructed of darkly tinted Plexiglass walls. To the left there was an orange hot-air balloon. Directly in front of him, Alex saw a huge mock-up of the Statue of Liberty. All of these stations belonged to the drug companies, which not only poured hundreds of thousands of dollars into their marketing booths on the exhibition floor, but also supported millions of dollars' worth of research with related symposiums at the convention.

The escalator reached the bottom and Alex stepped off. The plush red carpet felt good as he strode toward the right side of the floor, where he knew the publishers' aisle would be. Alex liked to begin his first tour of the convention floor with the books. The publishers' aisle had the look and feel of a book bazaar. The largest booth was actually a fair-size bookstore without walls, but with several large shelves and floor displays. From there on, the individual publishers set up smaller booths packed with books. Alex was always amazed at the sheer volume of books for sale. In his first years of practice, he would come to this convention and wind up spending a full two days wandering from bookstall to bookstall selecting dozens of books, most sent home by mail, but many of which he would have to lug back with him. Alex read every one.

Over the years, though the number of books published grew, the number Alex took home from the convention fell to almost none. He interpreted this not as a measure of the quality of the books or their relevance to his work, but more as a measure of his diminishing enthusiasm for dwelling on the major problems written about in books. It seemed to him that the fundamental problems of simple human decency were the ones that went begging.

Still, the book bazaar lured him. Here was a book on the genetics of mental illness. Here was a book about living with schizophrenia in the family. Here was a history of medicine. Here was a book on psychiatric disorders in children. Here was a book on the philosophy of psychiatry. Alex stood still in the middle of the aisle, staring at the cover of a book on *The Diseased Brain*, and, after a moment, understood why he was drawn to the books first. The entire convention represented mental functioning of a very high order. To turn the grim business of mental illness into a carnival required a high degree of intelligence. But of all that was going on here, the books represented the most concentrated mental function.

Alex was astounded and ultimately lured by the supreme act of consciousness, which a book represented at the highest level. Books on the mind were, to him, the most astounding: a mind turned in on itself, able not only to consider its functioning, but, amazingly, also to consider certain of its own functions as abnormal. It was one thing for the mind to examine a broken leg or a sick heart. But for the very instrument of examination to step back and examine itself! If for no other reason, this was why Alex was a psychiatrist. All other medicine could be reduced to mechanics. Not psychiatry, which forced the soul to the mirror and pried open its eyes.

Once through the books, which now took Alex only an hour or two, he stepped up his pace. About a third of the booths were manned by drug company salespeople, men and women who were trained not only to sell, but to carry on informed conversation with physicians about the drugs they were selling. The larger companies, with the heavily prescribed major psychiatric drugs, competed by means of huge, dramatic displays. They were not competing with different versions of the same drug, but with different drugs that might be used to treat the same problem. The stars of the show were the major antipsychotic drugs and tranquilizers. These were followed by the antidepressants, antianxiety drugs, and antiseizure drugs.

Some of the drug companies were there to entertain as well as sell. They accomplished this by showing films or videotapes of what their drugs could do, hence the minitheater set up by one and the array of lounge chairs with personal TV screens set up by another.

One company had constructed a miniature electronic classroom. Psychiatrists sat down to a computer screen and answered tricky diagnostic questions.

Alex already knew about all of the drugs from his religious reading of the journals. But he made sure to stop at each booth, nod pleasantly to the salesperson, and grab one of the pens or other trinkets being given away. Trick or treat for psychiatrists: About two-thirds of the booths gave something away, usually a pen with the company or hospital logo printed on it. Some gave away note pads, paperweights, or cassette tapes of lectures. Generally, the salesperson would try to engage the physician in conversation, hoping to snag a new order. To get away fast with a trinket the trick was to make and break eye contact as quickly as possible, to smile and say something nice without actually giving the salesperson a chance to ask you a question. Alex collected as much of the junk as he could on one or two passes through the hall. His kids loved the pens and the pads with the drug company logos on them.

Alex stopped at a drug company display for a famous antidepressant. A stage had been erected about ten feet above the floor, and two mimes were going through a stunted, slow-motion dance as if a heavy ceiling were lowering itself on them. Alex watched them for several minutes, then chuckled, grabbed a handful of blue pens out of an unguarded box on a table near the stage, and walked on.

Several private hospitals had booths, hoping not only to alert psychiatrists to their existence for possible referrals, but also to recruit them. Not to be outdone, several state departments of mental health had booths, too. Alex's state did not. Psychiatric residencies were down, and there was a shortage of psychiatrists nationwide. Despite the shortage, psychiatry was still one of the lowest paid medical specialties.

This year there were about a dozen companies that sold computerized brain-imaging machines. The subject sat in a chair and was fitted with a helmet—some looked like space helmets, some like football helmets with wires, some like wire-mesh bird's nests. The helmet picked up electrical impulses from the brain and sent the information to the computer, which printed out a "map" of brain activity in bright colors. The computer could be programmed to deliver a series of smaller maps showing the brain in action as various mental stimuli were applied.

Alex knew this was an extremely promising area of research. The array of rainbow colors filling in the outline of a brain might not look different to the untrained eye, but there were distinct differences among people with various diagnoses. A manic-depressive brain had different colors in different places and proportions than a schizophrenic brain—which, in turn, delivered a strikingly different map from that of a "normal" person. The brain maps were new, hard evidence that something physical was going on in the brains of mentally ill people. Alex knew, however, that although the current thrust of psychiatry was to establish that mental illness was a physical process and treat it as such, we really were not ready to completely acknowledge that the machinery of the intellect, and perhaps even the soul, was vulnerable to physical forces. We still wanted to make it into choices between good and evil, God and the Devil, will and weakness.

As for the scientific workshops and seminars and lectures, it was the same for Alex as with the books—a bewildering load of information, all of it solid and good, but just too much of it. Going over the program was an exercise in frustration. There were so many he would like to attend, but it was impossible to be in four places at once, which is what he would have had to do if he were to go to all the meetings that interested him.

So he usually wound up going to the "new research reports." Alex did not want to be seduced by any new hopes, yet it was refreshing to sit in a room and hear someone talk about psychiatry as if it were a solvable series of problems. In one room Alex heard the declaration that within our lifetimes we would see the complete genetic mapping of the brain, and that it would be a relatively short step from there to correcting all genetic defects, including those responsible for mental illness. Alex wondered if we would then see the elimination of mental illness, as well as most other diseases, or, instead, the opening of prebirth boutiques where those who could afford it would "order up" superperfect children, while those who couldn't would still take their chances in the genetic bingo game.

Aside from the drug company and serious psychiatric technology exhibits, most of the remaining booths were for various forms of psychiatric snake oil, albeit some of it highly accomplished technically: the vibrating lounge chairs connected to giant TV screens that lullabied your anxieties away with soft music and boring images of sunsets and birds flying along the beach or coasting on thermal currents in the mountains, the isolation chambers that took away your anxiety by depriving you of all sensation, the lights that relaxed away your anxieties, the furniture that cured madness because it was made of wood . . . the nutritional supplements . . . the biofeedback machines. . . .

There were psychiatric management firms that promised to remake a physician's life by supplying steady work in temporary situations—usually filling in for other psychiatrists on vacation, or filling in odd hours at clinics and in emergency rooms. In return, the physician did not have to worry about managing a practice and could take six weeks of vacation a year. Whatever they called it, it was just a fancy name for psych-temps. Have M.D. will travel. A medical day laborer: here comes the patient, what drug do you give 'em, sign off, and so long.

Alex knew that this kind of arrangement suited many physicians. Psychiatry seemed to have more than its share of drifters. An internist or surgeon could settle down in one place, build up a practice, and never leave. With psychiatrists, it didn't seem to work that way. Doc was one of the very few psychiatrists Alex knew who had practiced in the same place for more than five or six years. Did this say something about the breed, or was it a symptom of the general assault on the profession itself? When Doc started out, it was possible for a psychiatrist to set up a private practice, same as an internist or surgeon or GP. You were affiliated with the local hospital and you saw patients from the same socioeconomic groups as the internists and surgeons.

Over the past decade or so, this kind of arrangement had become more and more difficult to manage. Mainly because third-party payments were being withdrawn from psychiatry. As general medical-surgical services grew more expensive, insurance payments more or less kept pace. But as psychiatry grew more expensive, insurance companies reduced coverage. The same middle-class patients who were the bread and butter of a general medical practice were barred from psychiatry. Your choices were to either accept the slim pickings from the middle class or build a practice among the rich. Or get a job in the public sector, treating the sick in clinics, county centers, and state hospitals.

Alex had chosen the public path because, he felt, it freed him to practice medicine without worrying about the business of running a private practice.

Alex always stopped by the government booths: The National Institute of Mental Health, the Navy, the National Institute on Alcohol Abuse and Alcoholism. . . . He was always surprised to see the federal government represented. As a physician he was trained to examine an organism for signs of disease. In his case, as a psychiatrist, he looked for signs of mental disease, of dysfunctions in thought and deed. So when a single organism exhibited contradictory impulses, it was a warning sign. The fact that the government which supported so much valuable research and dissemination of knowledge was the same organism that was cutting funds for medical and social services while building more and bigger weapons of destruction perplexed him. The Navy was known to be one of the best places for a physician to practice medicine.

Insurance companies, HMOs, and medical management firms were there, too. So they had let the enemy in. The same people who were limiting coverage for psychiatric illness were represented, maybe in hopes that some kind of truce could be forged, or that what we really had was a problem in communication; that if we found out more about them and they found out more about us, we would all acknowledge that we were fine fellows and the problem would dissolve: they would stop eliminating coverage of psychiatric treatment.

[2]

"Dr. Greco, hello!"

The hand touching his arm woke Alex from his reverie.

"Fran Channing? You remember?"

"Of course, Mrs. Channing. Forgive me."

Fran was one of four people at the Family Organization booth. Alex scanned the literature on the table between him and Fran. *We Are Family* was the message on one pamphlet. *Mental Illness Is Everybody's Business* announced another. *Who Are the Mentally Ill?* yet another asked, and then answered: *We are your children, your brothers and sisters, your mothers and fathers. . . . One in four families is touched by severe mental illness.*

"Are you enjoying the convention?" Fran asked.

"Well . . . uhhh . . . I've been to a lot of these." Alex stammered.

"This is my first one. We always have a booth at them, though. Oh, are you going to the state capitol tomorrow?"

Alex looked puzzled.

"Well, let me tell you what's happening. The state budget is coming up. The governor wants to cut the mental health budget by 30 percent. He has refused to even grant an audience to anyone who argues against this. All he says is the money must come from either the mental health budget or the money for the blind, aged, and disabled. Imagine that!"

Alex shook his head.

"We're chartering buses and marching on the capitol," Fran said.

"This is not—" Alex started to say.

"We don't live here, but we're joining our members who do," Fran said. "There'll be buses here at eight."

"I'll check my schedule,"Alex nodded, and started backing away from the table. Fran smiled and turned to someone else who was approaching the booth. Alex felt suddenly free, and so he walked away.

At the end of the aisle, he stopped cold. There were various service booths set up, including a job-placement clearinghouse. There sitting at one of the tables, his head in one of the listing books, was George Konopski, the psychiatrist from the V-unit.

Alex understood. Konopski was one of the best psychiatrists at the hospital, one of the best Alex had ever known. Of course he would be looking for another job. Lately, Konopski had come under increasing pressure from Sam Akbar to perform a "courtesy" evaluation on Linus Dillinger. The "courtesy" was to the egos in the state attorney's office.

As he rode the escalator up to the exits, Alex became aware of a damp wave of anguish pressing at his back, and felt it subside as he rose into the clearer, brighter air of the entrance hall. He decided he would go to the demonstration. Perhaps what was needed was to reduce the entire array of frustrations and catastrophes to the elegance of a street brawl.

18 _____

[1]

More than twenty-four hours later, Alex waited in the hotel bar for George Konopski, whom he had called, and tried to let the images of the day march through his mind and into oblivion.

The sprawling lawn of the capitol building, baking under the inland-valley sun, was taken over by thousands of demonstrators. They were not only from the Family Organization, but from every social and professional organization that was involved in care for the mentally ill, including the mentally ill themselves. There were psychiatrists, psychologists, social workers, welfare workers, psych techs, nurses, and therapists. Unlike the convention of psychiatrists, this was a multicolored mob. Were it not for the placards, it could have been a city park jammed with about five or six times the number of people it was designed to accommodate. And children. And old folks. It was a people's march, after all, and that meant T-shirts and three-piece suits, white shirtsleeves glaring in the sun

152

and red dresses, blue jeans disappearing inside cowboy boots and fat ladies fanning themselves under oak trees.

The monitors did a good job, Alex thought. Mental patients every one, and for once the frowns that seemed to come naturally stood them well. Alex remembered the chill he had felt looking into the baby face of one of the monitors in the hallway outside a politician's office: a young man, perhaps twenty-two, chronic paranoid schizophrenic. Under control, mostly. Or in remission. Almost. When the word passed down through the crowd that not only would the governor not grant an audience to a delegation of the demonstrators, but that the man wasn't even in the city that day, the young monitor's face had screwed up into a grimace and he had muttered, "Just give me ten minutes alone with him. That's all I need."

The rally speeches outside the capitol were the usual expressions of indignant outrage by the politicians and anguish by the victims of the politicians.

Alex ordered a drink. Konopski was late, had, in fact, a history of being late.

And then the placards. There had been hundreds of them, but Alex remembered only a few: *Lives Are at Stake. The System Is Ill! Cut Bombers, Not People! Are We Going to Support Human Need, or Human Greed?*

Some of the signs were lengthy descriptions of the bearer's plight: *I was stricken schizophrenic 13 years ago and I am living on the street and . . .*

Or, *My children and I have no place to go. I cannot get a job. I am mentally ill.*

Initially, there was an infectious exuberance about the scene. This was democracy in action, and there was something hopeful and wonderful about this communion of grievances. But as the day wore on, Alex lost the exuberance. The assumption of the crowd was that if only the governor knew what they knew, and if only the man knew how earnest they were about wanting what they wanted for their loved ones and for themselves—and they were here to tell him—then his mind would be changed.

The governor knew all he had to know, Alex realized; knew, in fact, as much as anyone in the crowd. And this was a governor who was known as a "good" man, a "caring" man, a man whose name had come up as a presidential candidate, described as the great hope of the people who wanted to restore social services after more than a decade of neglect. A man who had roused many crowds over these same issues. He was the man who had left town. He was the man who had presided over the loss of over a billion dollars in health-care funds over the last decade, the man whose proposed budget would eliminate eight clinics that cared for the severely mentally ill, close a state hospital, and slash funds for children's health services. He was the man who wanted to build two new prisons.

Still no Konopski. Alex ordered a second drink.

What Alex remembered most vividly was the way the Channing woman held on to her enthusiasm and determination throughout the day. She kept her brow high and her back straight and went through the motions, from bus to capitol steps to politicians' offices, with never a hint that she believed this whole thing was any less than an expression of some kind of power. She was a warrior, and that was good, because she had herself a battle.

But while the demonstrators felt they were taking hills and small villages, there were rooms in the capitol where decisions were being made that would simply eliminate entire campaigns, just wipe battlefields off the map, and whole armies with them, regardless of whether they were winning or losing, and shake the human refuse on to another, more crowded theater of operations, into the jails or the streets.

What the day had been, Alex decided finally, was a convocation of refugees: patients, parents, relatives, social workers, psychologists, psychiatrists, techs, nurses—all of them crying under the sun, victims of a war of attrition.

Alex saw Konopski coming and felt relieved to see the familiar face from home. Alex hoped George had rotten luck at the placement service. Konopski slapped his hand on the other psychiatrist's shoulder.

"I see you started without me, Alex."

"You bet I did. I knew that's the way you would have wanted it."

They ordered a round. Alex felt an alcohol fog moving into his brain, but he still noticed that Konopski was watching him, as if trying to see if what he was hiding was showing.

"Look, George, I've got an idea that'll save us. Get us out of Bedloe before the you-know-what gets into the air conditioning."

"What air conditioning?"

"Right! That's what I mean! Look . . . here's what we do. We buy one of those brain-imaging computers. You know what I mean?"

Konopski nodded.

"We go to Hawaii, California, Arizona—anywhere there's a lot of foreign tourists swarming around—set up a little private practice."

Konopski forced a smile. "Ouch! Couldn't we talk about something a little more pleasant, like serial murder?"

Setting up private practice was a dead giveaway that this was a joke. If anyone knew how much George Konopski winced at the very mention of private practice it was Alex, who had hired the man from the wreckage of a twelve-year disaster of one.

"We take out ads in all the tourist magazines: GET A PICTURE OF YOUR BRAIN! UNDERSTAND YOUR MIND! Foreign tourists love that stuff. Charge 'em a thousand bucks for a complete workup. We'll pay for the machine the first month! Whatta ya say?"

"Count me in."

Konopski wrapped both hands around his drink and raised it to his mouth. Alex did the same.

[2]

That night, Alex's dream pursued him through the shroud pulled over his senses by the alcohol.

It was the same dream that had haunted him for months, in which he is the first Psychiatrist General of the United States of America, making rounds from coast to coast.

As the dream begins, Alex is standing in the fragrant shade of a tree in front of a huge clean white stucco building on a hill. Barely moving air rustles the thick leaves of the tree and slaps the crisp red, white, and blue canvas of the flag against the top of the pole in front of him. The same air has a balmy gentleness as it caresses his skin. He hears the sound of children playing carelessly, happily in a schoolyard across the street.

Now he is inside the building. The receptionist, a lovely blond nurse, smiles warmly.

Alex asks her the first question: "Is everyone taken care of?"

Alex knows she will not lie.

"Yes, Doctor," the nurse answers.

"Those who cannot take care of themselves, are they taken care of?" he asks, trying to be more specific.

"Of course, Doctor."

"Those whose minds are tied in knots? Are they taken care of? Those who don't know their names? Those who don't know what day this is, or what a day is? Are they taken care of?"

"Everyone is taken care of, Doctor," the nurse answers patiently.

"Nurse, what about those whose minds are twisted by sickness and pain and who cause pain in others? Are they taken care of?"

"Yes, Doctor."

"The children who are abandoned, or abused?"

The nurse nods reassuringly and closes her blue eyes reverently.

"And the families torn apart by madness? What about them?"

"We do the best we can, Doctor, for everyone," she says in a soothing whisper, aware of his anguish.

"See for yourself, Doctor," the nurse says cheerfully.

The doors open into a large, sunlit dayroom—which is so clean it sparkles. The room is brightly decorated with hanging plants, paintings that look like they might have been done by children or patients, and posters of animals. The room is deserted. There is a nurse's station in the middle, also deserted.

"Where is everyone?"

"Outside, of course. It's such a lovely day. Nobody wants to be inside, Doctor. Come, I'll show you."

Alex blinks and is in the middle of a park. There are people dressed in red, white, and blue all around him. Small groups of a dozen or so are hiking here and there across the park. A group of men is milling around on a baseball diamond off to the side. In a grove of trees at the top of a hill two or three dozen people are lying in the gentle grass courageously attempting yoga stretches. A group of small children sits under an oak tree and listens to a fairy tale told by an older patient who believes the story is true.

A group of patients march by, heartily enjoying their walk, which is led by a smiling pair of young women. Alex watches them hike across the meadow. The breeze caresses him again, blows the little tendrils of his hair around his temples, and then moves on to stir the grass and the leaves in the trees.

"This is an extraordinary institution."

"No, not really, Doctor. Every hospital is pretty much a duplicate of this one."

"Everywhere? Every state? Every city?"

"Yes, Doctor." The nurse looks surprised that he doesn't know.

"Who pays for all this?"

"This is the richest country in the world, Doctor. You should know that. Silly question."

"Ha!" he explodes, sarcastically.

The nurse takes a deep breath, and shakes her head as she lets out the breath.

"Silly man. You should know. You designed the program! Don't you remember?"

It is time to travel. Alex is high above the ground, flying over the city with the angelic nurse. It is early Sunday morning, he can tell from the super-thick bundles of fat newspapers waiting on street-corners. The syrupy, slightly phony songs of electronic church bells drift up to him.

Superdoctor scans the streets for those in need. The same power-ful eyes that can diagnose illness at a glance now train themselves on the dark places in doorways, on alleys, benches, and trash piles.

From the air, Superdoctor can scan the city and look into the hearts of its homes. He sees children beaten and drugged and raped. He sees the seeds of madness start to sprout in young and vibrant minds. He sees old people chattering nonsense in their loneliness, fearing but hungering for death. He sees that same appetite for oblivion in young people taking drugs.

"We're not perfect," the nurse says, anticipating his concern. "But we're not savages, either. We try our best. Everyone we know about is taken care of."

And now Alex finds that he has a hint of that same appetite for oblivion himself. The nurse sees the disturbed look on his face and knows that he is hiding something.

"Do you know of one, Doctor?"

Alex tenses. He leans over to her, cups his hand between his mouth and her ear and whispers the name.

"Carmen Greco. Is she cared for?"

The nurse concentrates, looks back and flips through her memory file, and then shakes her head with sincere concern. "No, Doctor, she's not. I'm sorry."

Alex knows what the nurse is going to say next, and he doesn't want to hear it.

"But you know, Doctor, I think she'll be getting in touch with you," the nurse says with an efficient smile.

There is the house. And Alex doesn't want to, but he is coming in for a gentle landing right in front of it, touching the ground near the white picket fence with the neat flower arrangements bordering it. Beyond the fence there is a fashionably overgrown yard, and in the middle of the yard a white two-story colonial. The front door is open. Inside the house, Alex Greco's house, the phone is ringing.

Alex feels surrounded by dread. He wishes the nurse would answer the phone, but the nurse is no longer in the dream. The house is empty, the dream is empty, and in these moments before he awakens, the world is empty except for Alex and the telephone.

19

[1]

Riding the bus back to the convention, Fran Channing had asked Alex if he would consent to speak at the next meeting of the Family Organization. He agreed in what he believed was a moment of guilt and confusion. Alex felt drawn to the Family Organization, and Fran's invitation took advantage of his confusion to reach through his resistance to his own need.

Alex told Fran he would do what he could to improve hospital policy toward the Family Organization. Fran and the others on the bus told him that there were some specific reforms which other chapters of the Organization had implemented at other hospitals and all of which resulted in improvements in care. Alex agreed and promised to try to open doors for them at Bedloe.

A few days after he returned from the convention, Alex visited Sam Akbar. "I have some proposals," he said, "which I believe will improve the level of care here."

Ignoring Sam's grimace, Alex went on to propose that family

159

members be allowed into the hospital in four ways. First, he wanted to loosen some of the visiting restrictions to make it easier for the units to hold holiday and birthday celebrations. That would raise morale and allow relatives contact with staff in an informal, casual setting.

Second, Alex wanted to allow family members to sit in on treatment-team meetings when the staff of each unit met to discuss progress and treatment options for individual patients.

Third, Alex wanted to invite family members to sit in on meetings at which policies for the entire hospital were supposedly discussed and set. Alex knew the meetings were mostly a debating society. Akbar made all the decisions behind his office doors, keeping whatever counsel he wanted.

Sam said that having a barbecue or holiday party every now and then would be just fine. "Good press" were his exact words. But he flatly rejected any involvement of the family members in treatment or policy meetings. As Alex had figured he would.

"What's the fourth thing? You said there were four," Sam barked impatiently.

"Yes. Well, the parents would like to meet with you personally."

"What the hell for? Just to ask for these things all over again? I've already said, no way."

"Well, you see they've been working on a survey of care at the hospital. All the family members with relatives here have been sent a questionnaire. In a week or so they'll have the results. I think it will be a valuable report from a different point of view. I intend to give it a very serious examination."

"You do that, Alex. But why do they want to see me?"

"I imagine they want to talk to you about it face to face. You know, establish some kind of personal rapport."

Sam grunted. "Yeah, that bullshit."

"They've done good things at other hospitals."

"Hmmmph. Well, I suppose I could meet with them. Have them call my secretary."

The Family Organization's meeting with Akbar came on a day when Alex was at the state capital on routine matters with the state director of mental health. When he returned to the hospital the next day, Akbar was away and all Alex could find out was that the meeting had been short.

The next day, Sam was still out of town. Alex asked Sam's secretary if he could have a copy of the Family Organization survey of care at the hospital. The secretary said she knew of no such document.

That evening was the Family Organization meeting. As Alex was trying to get out the door from under his wife's busily grooming fingers, adjusting his collar and brushing his jacket, the phone rang. Maria's and Alex's eyes met, and then Maria trailed her hand on her husband's arm for as long as she could as he walked away to answer it.

"Hi, Dad. Hi, Dad. This is your daughter, Carmen, Dad."

[2]

The church basement was packed. Fran mused that the Family Organization might have to find a larger meeting place soon, and she knew that was good.

The meeting was late getting started and people were getting restless. She had arranged for Alex to speak first, but he had not arrived yet. Fran wanted to talk to him before he gave his report. Among other things, she wanted to thank him for setting up the organization's meeting with Sam Akbar. By now most members knew all about the incident.

When Fran saw Alex come into the packed basement, she hurried to make her way over to him.

"Dr. Greco," she said as they shook hands. "I'm glad you made it here tonight."

"I'm sorry I'm late, Mrs. Channing." He seemed glad to see her, relieved, Fran thought, as she walked with him through the crowd toward the front of the room. But also tired, drained of color and of some essence deeper than color.

"Doctor, I want you to know that after our meeting with Sam Akbar we really understand what you're up against." Her voice cracked with emotion as she told him about the meeting. When presented with the survey of care at the hospital, the superintendent had smiled and issued a theatrical sigh. He seemed to be nervously eyeing his watch as he stammered through a speech about looking into these problems. Then his phone rang.

Moments later, the delegation found themselves walking to their cars. Fran felt a cardboard heaviness in her gut, and was too angry and disgusted even to visit her son.

Fran left Alex's side and went to her seat in the front row. But Alex was still standing where she'd left him, following her with his eyes, nodding.

Then he was at the podium, being introduced by Anita Sansone. As the polite applause died down, Alex touched the lectern for support and looked out over the crowded room. When he had come to the meeting three months previously, the room had been less than half full. Now every seat was taken and there were people standing along the walls.

He shuffled his papers.

Most of the faces were smiling politely.

Alex could feel the sweat beading on his brow. The papers were sticking to his fingers.

He took a deep breath. A phone rang in the hallway and he felt himself jump, and wondered if anyone noticed.

"Uhh . . . I brought a prepared speech, with statistics. But . . . I suddenly realize that you people know these facts and issues at least as well as I do."

Alex saw that people frowned or squinted to focus more sharply on this foolish psychiatrist in the front of the room.

"So I'm going to put my speech aside for the moment . . . and improvise."

The phone rang again. Alex didn't jump this time, but something broke inside him, and he felt himself bow slightly at the lectern. He heard people clearing their throats. He heard someone get up and run to answer the phone.

"I have a dream I want to tell you about. I wish I could say this was the kind of dream politicians say they have, a dream meaning a fervently desired goal. But that's not what I mean. I mean a story played back to me by my brain when I am asleep.

"The dream tortures me.

"It always begins the same way: I am standing in front of a beautiful building, and it's a balmy spring day. I walk into the building and I am met by a beautiful blond nurse."

There was a titter of laughter in the crowd and Alex looked up sheepishly and smiled.

"It is a mental hospital.

"I am astounded by what I see at the mental hospital. In this mental hospital I dream, everyone is cared for with warmth and decency. Everyone—no matter how severely ill, no matter how unattractive their illness.

"In the dream I keep asking . . . is everyone taken care of? And the kind nurse always answers 'Yes, Doctor' . . . or . . . 'Of course, Doctor' . . . or . . . 'We do the best we can, Doctor.'

"And at every step of the way, as this nurse leads me through the hospital, my anxiety and . . . my pain intensify because it is so beautiful. It works so well. At every turn I find another area in which the care is humane and effective. Patients are outside. It's such a nice day the wards have been emptied. They are playing games, telling stories, singing songs.

"Let me hasten to assure you this dream is not about a world where mental illness had been eradicated. There are patients in this hospital who have been there, or will be there, for their entire lives.

"But then the really painful part comes, when I find out that this is not an extraordinary institution. The nurse tells me that every hospital in the land is a virtual duplicate of this one.

"And then she tells me that I should know, because I designed the program!

"I'm not taking any great credit, nor do I in the dream. Any one of you could design this system of care for the mentally ill. We all know what decent, humane care for the sick is, and we all know when it isn't provided.

"And it isn't happening now, in our country. That is what makes this dream such torture for me. I wake up from it and I know that our entire system of care for the mentally ill is a bedlam.

"Our public hospitals, mental hospitals and medical-surgical hospitals, are tents of misery and shame. Our city streets are awash with suffering and brutality.

"I am afraid for us, because the sight of this has not shamed us into action.

"At the end of my dream, the nurse answers the wonder and the pain on my face by telling me, 'We're not perfect, but we're not savages, either. Everyone we know about is taken care of.'

"Today, we cannot make that statement."

Alex looked around at the faces in front of him. They seemed to want more from him, as if they knew there was more to the dream that he wasn't telling them. But Alex didn't know how to tell them about the ringing phone and the empty house.

Well, just say it. He opened his mouth and started to confess . . . but nothing came out. Alex knew if he took that step he might collapse totally. It was bad enough he had thrown away his prepared speech and delivered this rambling drivel. Now what was he going to do?

There was some polite, tentative applause, which quickly died down when Alex looked up and started to open his mouth.

"Thank you," he said, barely above a whisper. Then he started again, "As I was making my way to the podium here, Fran Channing said to me, 'Dr. Greco, now we know what you're up against.' "

Alex sighed deeply.

"But I must tell you something. I must confess to you that I know, and have known all along, what *you* are up against."

Fran watched Alex's eyes, which she could tell he was forcing to keep wide open against a flood of emotion that wanted to close them. The room was as silent as a vacuum.

"I am the father of a mentally ill child. My daughter has schizophrenia and is currently living in a marginal situation, alternating between the streets, her maternal grandmother's house, and a single-room-occupancy hotel about three hundred miles from here. She is in agony. There is nothing I can do for her. . . ."

Alex could go no further. He wished he could stop his breathing, because it was so loud to him he was sure everyone could hear it.

The silence expanded, swelled until no one could stand it. Alex bowed his head slightly, and the room erupted in applause. People were coming up to shake his hand and talk to him. "Thank you, Doctor," they were all saying. Fran Channing was among them, smiling broadly.

"You cannot imagine what it feels like," Fran said, "when we find a doctor who is on our side."

We tend to think of healing as the closing of a wound. But some things are broken in the closed position, and healing opens them. Alex felt buoyed by the Family Organization people gathering around him. But among all the accepting voices there was one speaking to him from inside his own heart, and it told him this: *Alex Greco, M.D., you are not doing enough.*

20

Breakfast was a clamorous time at Bedloe State Hospital. Before the first patients sat down to their bacon and eggs and toast, the last in a series of trucks delivering food to the loading dock behind the kitchen would be coughing smoke as it chugged up the hill around back. Inside the kitchen, plates crashed and silverware clanged. Arguments broke out among the kitchen staff, though only rarely among the patient-helpers. Toast was burned and milk was spilled and backdoors were opened to let out the heat and the noise and the tension.

There was a small cafeteria connected to the kitchen, but it was mostly for staff. Patients rarely used it. Each ward had its own small dining room, to which food was trucked. Smaller hospitals might get by with a central cafeteria, but Bedloe, even at one-fifth capacity, was still too big to schedule all its units for one facility three times a day. So every morning the psych techs rousted sleepy patients from their beds to get them to their dining area as close as possible to when the food arrived from the kitchen. Tables were set optimistically, with napkins and knives, and the staff braced themselves.

The dining rooms hummed and buzzed and crashed along. An occasional piece of food flew through the air, launched by an obscenity and greeted by several more upon landing. Arguments and fights broke out with slightly more frequency than in a high-school cafeteria, but with slightly less damage done to most of the combatants. Although the patients made a terrible mess, there was more physical distress caused by wild bacteria in the food than by wild patients. And there was more laughter than crying, more eating than arguing, more joking than cursing. On most mornings, anyway.

After the patients left, hospital workers would attack the mess, but the real cleaning would not come until after supper. Until then, clean enough was as clean as anything got.

Breakfast marked a new day, if not a new life, a time of opportunities, a time for staff to clean up areas of the unit that could not be cleaned when patients were around. It was a time when, in the quiet of the empty ward, good work could be done.

Doc, for one, was always torn between accompanying patients to breakfast or staying behind to finish up paperwork. The paperwork lost the battle most of the time.

George Konopski usually accompanied residents of the V-unit to breakfast, because the staff needed all the hands they could get.

D-7 always arrived late and ate cold food, a fact that was not lost on the kitchen staff. Dean Lester rarely ate breakfast with his patients. Instead he remained in the unit and caught up on his morning soap operas and talk shows. This fact was not lost on Alex, who chose breakfast as the time to summon the psychiatrist to his office and fire him.

Alex told Lester the ward was a disgrace to medicine and a blight on the hospital, and that he wanted him out by the end of the day.

Lester's face hardened. "You'll hear from my lawyer," he said.

"Well," Alex said, "actually, I've already notified your lawyer that not only am I dismissing you, but notifying the medical quality board, too. You'll receive copies of the letter."

That was it as far as Lester was concerned.

Now Alex had to tell Sam Akbar. He figured he might as well do it on the same blast of adrenaline, so he waited only five minutes after Lester walked out.

"I want you to know that I fired Dean Lester, effective immediately."

Akbar lurched forward. "You what?"

"Fired him. I don't want him on my medical staff."

Alex did not allow Sam any room to maneuver. "I've already got enough on Lester to bring him up on charges before the state medical quality board. I've written his attorney a letter to that effect. If we hold on to him, it's not going to look too good when the accreditation committee shows up."

Akbar's eyes flared like a cornered animal's. But there was nothing he could do. Not yet.

21 _____

[1]

Without any prompting from Doc or Rosey or anyone, Wendy celebrated her birthday in July by dumping Bert. She took an early lunch one day and got to the deserted office half an hour ahead of schedule and left a "Dear Bert" letter.

Meanwhile, back in Wilson Cottage, Doc was worried about Lily Speere. In her therapy sessions Lily was starting to reveal a depth to her depression that surprised Doc. Wendy, who had resisted any decrease in medication, had been right. He decided to put off the decision whether or not to reduce her medication.

Zelda Glover, killer of two husbands, gave Wendy a pillow with Wendy's likeness embroidered on it.

Greta Lampson was getting worse. Doc came back from visiting her in the infirmary and just shook his head. "She's losing weight," he muttered to Wendy. "She refuses to eat. They're feeding her with a tube, but you know that doesn't do the job. She's undernourished.

169

Her burns aren't healing. You know what she said to me? She said, 'It doesn't matter what you do. I'm going to win.' "

Doc and Wendy were keeping a close eye on Ethel Flynn since eliminating her medications when her pregnancy became evident. She had been on very light meds, anyway, so they did not expect any serious decompensation. And they saw none, unless holding hands with Dr. Rose could be considered a symptom.

For his part, Rosey's main contribution to the life of the unit, aside from his time spent with Ethel Flynn and a handful of other patients, was to raise the noise level of arguments about patients' medications in treatment-team meetings.

After one particularly energetic disagreement, Doc and Wendy took Rosey aside after the meeting.

Wendy started. "Okay, it's true that Doc and I get into some terrible fights because . . . if I believe in something I'll fight until my dying breath. And Doc feels very strongly about letting a patient have most of the control over whether they take their meds. He feels that if he lets them have control now, they'll pretty much be in control when they leave here. That sort of makes sense to me. They pretty much do what they want when they leave here anyway."

"I don't understand," Rosey said.

"You haven't told him what we really fight about, Wendy," Doc said with a smile.

Wendy grimaced. "Well, Doc tends to want the patients to get by with as little medication as possible. We usually fight about that, like when he wants to give a patient less medication and I want to give more. See . . . I . . . I see these patients at their worst. And . . . you gotta understand. . . ." she glanced at Doc again.

"Go ahead. I know what you're going to say and I want Dr. Rose to hear it."

"We've got a lot of patients in here who are borderline personalities. They love playing games. They love to play one person against another. That's my experience. They love to get the staff fighting among themselves. So they'll go in and see Doc and be real nice and say they'd like to get off their meds because it makes them feel so drowsy or something and they'll be real nice. But when they're around me, they're not always so nice. We had a guy in here, schizophrenic person, but he also had a borderline personality, I guess, because he loved to play games, too. He had hallucinations and he heard voices. The voices told him to stick things in his ears. Usually it was cigarette butts. He figured that was going to block out the voices. I gave this guy all sorts of medicine—by the capful—and he still had the problem. But he still went in for his session with Doc and asked to have his meds reduced!"

A broad smile played across Doc's face. "And I did it, too."

Wendy smiled, too. "Yes you did!"

"And, brother, did they hand it to me at the next treatment-team meeting!"

"Well," Wendy said, "you didn't have to pull cigarette butts out of this poor guy's ears all day long. He didn't even smoke. He'd scrounge the butts from the ashtrays and the other patients."

"Where is he now?" Rosey asked.

Doc looked at Wendy for the answer.

"Hmmm . . . that was Caldwell . . . . he went back to the county, I think. Yeah. That was a couple of years ago."

Then it was Doc's turn. "Rosey, there's a lot going on in the treatment of the mentally ill that I don't like and that you're right not to like. But, take it from an eyewitness, the quality of psychiatric care in general has improved tremendously, and a lot of that improvement is because of psychiatric medications. You know I spent part of my training at a state hospital—almost fifty years ago. We had some tranquilizers back then, too, barbiturates. They helped with some patients. But we also found ourselves using hydrotherapy. Why, we still have a hydrotherapy room here at Bedloe somewhere."

"What is that?"

"You had two hoses, one with hot water and one with cold. The patient was put in this sort of open-ended shower and sprayed with alternating hot and cold water."

"Water torture."

"Not at all. It worked. Sure there was a lot of screaming and protesting—but it calmed the patient down. And the only side effect was that the patient got clean. But we also had something called a cold-wet pack. The patient was wrapped fairly tightly in wet sheets. They couldn't move at all. It literally cooled people off—tranquilized them. People who had it described it as warming their bodies and giving them a real sense of security. It was not painful or uncomfortable in any way. But this has long gone out of existence and it's interesting to philosophize why." Doc looked at Rosey expectantly, giving him a chance to answer.

"The drugs came along and were aggressively marketed so they took over."

"Well, I guess you could say that. But look, it took two or three staff members to administer hydrotherapy. If you can do the same thing by giving a pill, you save time and money. Psychiatry is a pretty expensive specialty. The amount of money that's spent taking care of patients is enormous—it's such a chronic business. It's not like surgery. With an appendectomy you get sick in the morning and within a day your appendix is out. A few days later you're out of the hospital. Major surgeries like bypasses and cancer surgeries—it can be two or three weeks from diagnosis to discharge from the hospital. With chronic mental illness you have people spending years and years of their lives in the hospital. Sometimes their entire lives.

"One of the discouraging things about meds is that while antipsychotic medications are a great advance and really a great help in the treatment of advanced illness, not all patients respond reliably. Their hallucinations, delusions, and other symptoms are not always affected. They come to Bedloe State Hospital because they can't be maintained in community mental health centers or in board-and-care homes. So the patients we get here are sicker and stay longer.

"Our number of patients remains about the same because it's kept artificially low by means of a restrictive admissions policy. The state-hospital budget keeps shrinking. Our society has decided to rotate mentally ill people through the system rather than actually make a commitment to treat them or take care of them. So many go through here, we see them for awhile, then they are discharged prematurely to get sick again and wander through the system and the streets until they wind up back here. We see an endless parade of the sickest of the sick. There isn't a great deal of time we can spend face to face with a patient. So we do the best we can with what we have. Most of the time, that means psychoactive drugs. It's true we don't know precisely how they work. There are areas of the brain and certain functions we know they affect, but in most cases we can't draw a diagram of what's really going on, whether something's being repaired, replaced, turned off, turned on, turned up, or turned over! They don't always work, but we've got to try."

Doc wanted to let that sink in. He also wanted to look for signs of a response in his audience. He saw none, only an implacable and slightly defensive frown.

"It teaches you patience," Doc sighed, more to himself than to Rosey.

[2]

Doc tried to use his new patient, Bennett Ackerman, to demonstrate to Rosey how drugs could prepare the way for effective psychotherapy. Few of the psychiatrists at Bedloe stole enough time for more than brief psychotherapy sessions with their patients. Doc seemed to be able to steal more time than most. As happens in any undertaking the size of Bedloe State Hospital, it was a natural tendency for the staff to slide into a dull drudgery where only what absolutely must be done was ever attempted. There were so many bureaucratic duties that the institution valued more than therapy—such as paperwork—that most staff had to step outside normal procedure in order to perform any of the acts that might be described as fundamental to their profession. Doc was one who not only swam against the current, but also managed to drag several poor souls upstream along with him. He stole time for therapy by neglecting paperwork, coming in on Saturdays, or performing all bureaucratic drudgery in a mechanical, thoughtless, but speedy manner.

Of course, not all patients were "candidates" for therapy. Different physicians had different guidelines for making the distinction, but some of the patients were too ill for therapy. For some, judicious use of medications would enable them to benefit from therapy. For others, no amount of medication could calm them enough to enable them to carry on a coherent conversation.

A short man of about fifty years old, Bennett Ackerman had been a successful businessman, husband, and father, until one Sunday morning his wife of twenty-four years found him huddled in a corner of the garage behind some large boxes of old clothes. There was a note pinned to Bennett's shirt, written in his hand. "My head has been stolen," was scrawled across the paper in the disjointed, awkward script of a person writing in the dark or with his eyes closed.

Bennett Ackerman had been a jovial man given to practical jokes and hilarious stunts among his many friends, his wife had told the first in a long series of psychiatrists whose reports made up his file. But when Bennett failed to respond to the ministrations of the private psychiatric hospitals and his insurance coverage ran out, his wife moved swiftly to preserve the estate. After several months of legal maneuvers even she did not fully understand, she was the conservator of most of her husband's worldly goods, while the state was conservator of his body and mind. She had felt a twisting knot in her stomach when her attorney explained this procedure, and hastened to reassure her that this was the only way. After all, the insurance company had just dropped Bennett when his illness became too expensive, hadn't they? The society had constructed ways for corporations to back out of certain contracts and promises when they became too costly. She had the same right, the attorney explained.

So after a brief, unproductive stay at the county hospital, Bennett was transferred to Bedloe State Hospital. He was fortunate to come from a relatively rich and politically healthy county, so there was a bed all paid up for him.

So here was Bennett Ackerman, who already had been branded a lost soul, lost to his former gilded upper-middle-class life, lost to his wife and children, lost to himself. At least that's what the man's file suggested. Doc wondered. He was still, the file said, insisting that his head had been stolen. Doc couldn't wait to talk to this man. He had an idea, a plan, and the thought of it tickled him inside like a joke he knew was just right for a certain friend, like finding the perfect birthday present for a favorite child and hiding it until the moment of giving.

"Bennett," Doc began. "It says here you believe your head was stolen. Is that right?"

"Yes, Doctor."

"Well, Bennett, how is it that I can look at you and see a head on your shoulders, and speak to you, have you hear me, and speak back to me? I see a head with lips moving. You're talking to me."

Bennett had been through this many times, and Doc knew it, but he needed a place to start. If nothing else, going over this familiar ground would put Bennett at ease.

"Doctor, the people who stole my head are wizards. Maybe they're from another planet. That sounds crazy, I know. But wherever they're from, they know how to control minds. What they've done is, in place of my head, left a thought-projection screen. When you look at me, you see their projected thought-images of my head."

"I see. And when you look in the mirror?"

Bennett nodded happily. "You've got it, Doctor, I'm seeing the projected thought-image of my head, too. But I know it's not there. I know it's gone."

Doc knew what question he wanted to ask Bennett, but it wasn't time yet.

"Bennett, whenever a crime is committed, the police always look for a motive. We're kind of like detectives here, too. I can't think of a motive why these wizards would steal your head. Do you know why they would want to do that?"

Bennett nodded. "A sacrifice. They're very primitive wizards and they stole my head to make a sacrifice to their god."

"I see."

That was as far as Doc wanted to take it the first time. Bennett seemed content enough with the situation. He wasn't depressed, anxious, or agitated, so there was no pressure on Doc to deal with any behavioral problems. He could take his time and sort of sneak up on this man's craziness.

Besides, Doc had to prepare his "cure." That took some time and extra effort—mostly shopping around town.

When Doc had everything he needed, he knew he was ready to press Bennett a little harder.

"Bennett, I want you to tell me something. Do you promise to tell me the truth?"

Bennett Ackerman's eyes met Doc's for an instant. He frowned and answered, "Yes, Doctor."

"Okay. Good. Bennett, I want you to tell me how it felt when you lost your head."

Bennett looked at Doc again, then he looked away, tried to smile, and then looked down. He shook his head. Could it be that he had never been asked this question?

"It felt . . . bad."

"How did it feel bad? In what way? Painful? Fearful? Sick? How?"

"It didn't hurt, exactly. It felt . . . lonely. It felt . . . like I lost something."

"What did you lose, Bennett?"

Bennett seemed to sink his head even lower. His arms hung down on his lap, where his hands loosely clutched each other.

"All the things that were in my head. They're gone now."

"I see. Well, Bennett, there were some good things in your head, I suppose. Am I right?"

"Yes there were. Some wonderful things."

"I'll bet it was like losing a bunch of old scrapbooks, full of snapshots of your kids, or your mom and dad, or . . ."

Bennett rubbed his eyes and coughed.

"Would you like to have your head back, Bennett?"

Bennett shook his head.

"No, Doctor, that's impossible. They won't give it back. It's gone for good."

"It doesn't feel so good, not having a head, does it?"

Bennett shook his head, the one he didn't believe he had. And Doc knew that somewhere in Bennett's mind, residing in that missing head, was the knowledge that the head was present. But that knowledge was being held for ransom. Doc didn't know what the ransom was, but getting Bennett to admit that it hurt to lose the head, that there were good things in the head, was an important step, one that would be aided by Bennett's antipsychotic medication.

Why his head had been kidnapped could remain a mystery forever. It could be a microscopic mistake somewhere in the way Bennett's brain cells were organized. Maybe he'd had too much to drink one night and accidentally burned the wrong circuits. Or maybe the key contact points had simply deteriorated with age. Or perhaps some powerful passion within Bennett had forged this hallucination willfully, for some dark purpose. Or some light purpose. Bennett's brain could be playing an immense practical joke on itself.

Most likely, it was a little bit of all of the above. Doc accepted that situation. "A little bit of everything" he could work with. As long as there was a least a portion of the illness that was wired through the will, he could make some progress with psychotherapy. Even if that progress was only getting the patient to admit to his pain.

"That's all for today, Bennett."

Doc let him go. Even though he felt he had the "cure" for

Bennett's pain, he wanted to let Bennett live with it for awhile. He knew he was taking a chance. Bennett might be overcome with the grief and withdraw totally or attempt suicide. Doc doubted that would happen.

Bennett was fine for another week, though depressed and in mourning for the loss of his head. Doc figured that was long enough to wait, and so called his patient in for a session.

"Bennett," he got right to the point, "I think the people who stole your head are ready to give it back to you."

He watched Bennett for a reaction. The man just shook his head and continued to look dejected.

Doc reached behind him and grabbed a large round cardboard box. He placed the box on his desk, got up, and opened the box.

Out of the box, Doc took a large red cowboy hat. In place of the ribbon around the bowl of the hat, there were sewn into the hat a series of weights, so that when Doc lifted the hat, instead of weighing a pound, it weighed closer to three or four pounds.

Doc walked over to Bennett and placed the hat on his head. It fit snugly.

I guessed right, Doc congratulated himself.

Bennett sat up straight. He reached up and felt the brim of the hat.

"Bennett, how do you like your hat?"

"It's . . . it's . . ."

"Bennett, you're touching the hat. I want you to let your hand slide down from the hat to your ear."

Bennett followed Doc's directions.

"Now feel your cheek."

"It's . . . it's . . ."

"Move your head from side to side."

Bennett obeyed.

"Feel the weight? That's a real feeling. That's your head."

Bennett's face brightened. His head seemed to bob around, as he tested the new sensation of weight and substance.

"It's my head, I got it back. I feel it."

Doc exhaled a deep breath he had been holding for a long while.

"Yes, Bennett. You got your head back."

And there was Bennett, walking gaily around the unit with his big red cowboy hat.

"Is that all there is to it?" Rosey asked, later.

"Of course not," Doc answered. "I just borrowed a trick from a psychiatrist who did the same thing . . . two hundred years ago. Bennett's got a long way to go. Whatever prompted him to lose his head in the first place is still there. It's just resting now, in part thanks to his medication. The hat's kind of like a drug, too. It closes off part of the illness. We'll have to get into why he arranged to have his head stolen in the first place. That will take time, I think."

"How long?"

"Well," Doc smiled, "it could happen next session and he could all of a sudden look at his watch and say, 'Oh my, I'm late for dinner,' and jump right back into his life as if nothing ever happened. But I doubt it. Or, he could never go back. Look at him, he's perfectly happy with that hat. Whatever it was that sent him here, he may not want to ever go back."

Doc knew he was romanticizing Bennett Ackerman's illness, and that was supposed to be the first lesson you learned as a psychiatrist: There's nothing romantic about mental illness. Nothing proud or glorious or noble, no more than there is about cancer or heart disease or multiple sclerosis. Doc knew he was in dangerous territory. Psychoanalysis had a tendency to romanticize madness, to reduce it to themes, to give it meaning.

Doc had believed in those themes once, but now he generally scoffed at them. They were fine for stories, and they did come in handy for some psychotherapy. But mental illness was about as romantic as a bad bus accident and if there was any meaning in a smashed life, Doc didn't want to contemplate it.

Yet, in order to proceed as a psychiatrist and be more than a dispenser of medications, he had to somehow engage the patient in some kind of therapy. That meant engaging the patient's will. Was that the same as admitting that the patient's illness was willful?

No, Doc thought, that was nonsense. Mental illness didn't originate in the will, it preyed on the will, as it preyed on every other function of the brain. Doc knew that the patient's will might be an ingredient, even a necessary one, but it wasn't sufficient to cause the illness. Nor could the patient's will, alone, fight the disease and expect to win. You had to get help from outside—and that's what the physician was there for, that's what Doc was there for.

If the patient was fortunate enough to have any will left, psychotherapy could try to get its attention, throw it some kind of line, rescue as much as possible. Sometimes that could be quite a bit. Other times when you got the line out and pulled there just wasn't much left after the teeth of the disease had done their work.

Though Wendy and just about everyone else had their doubts, Doc believed there was a lot left in Bennett Ackerman.

[3]

Drugs could not penetrate the tangled mess of terror and anguish that was Mary Johnson's mind. Nor could Doc with his skills, nor Wendy with her muffins and picnics at the lake. As for the other staff of Wilson Cottage, the psych techs and nurses and therapists and psychologists had completely given up on her. Mary often sat motionless, peering out from behind her eyes with suspicion and palpable fear. She could be seen to bristle when anyone walked by, her body tensed and her eyes darted back and forth like two large, wet, black flies trapped inside her head.

If someone came too close, Mary would scream. Once in a while instead of screaming she would shield her face with her arms, stick her legs out and kick wildly. Often when someone came too close, Mary cried out like a hurt, cornered animal and flung herself on the person, clawing and slapping and biting. When this happened, the staff had no choice but to put her in the seclusion room. The usual procedure in Wilson Cottage was that when a patient became particularly unruly or became an actual physical threat to other patients or staff, he or she was asked to stop. If the patient did not stop the assaultive behavior, he or she was placed in a seclusion room for anywhere from fifteen minutes to several hours.

The Wilson Cottage staff did not like the seclusion room. While there were units at Bedloe that had all three or four of their seclusion rooms in use at any given time of the day or night, Wilson Cottage's three seclusion rooms were rarely used at all. In fact, one of them had been pressed into service as a storage room. The staff liked to try alternatives before putting a patient in seclusion. If the assaultive behavior occurred during the day, and there was enough staff, a psych tech might take the person for a walk on the park-like grounds of the hospital. The patients loved to go for walks, of course, especially those who did not have jobs that took them out of the ward for most of the day. Every now and then one or two of them would fake assaultive behavior just to go for a walk. Sometimes Wendy and another psych tech would take the entire unit for a walk.

But Mary Johnson not only did not respond to walks, she couldn't be taken on one. When a staff member approached her to take her for a walk she would cower, try to hide, or kick and scream. At a treatment-team conference, the staff decided that the young woman still feared the neighborhood boys were out there to abuse her. Doc wondered whether Mary Johnson even belonged in Wilson Cottage, her level of functioning was so low. The psychologist who had performed her initial evaluation in the Receiving Unit agreed that Mary was certainly very close to the minimum level of functioning required for a unit like Wilson Cottage.

Still, there was evidence of a higher level of functioning in her history. She had held a job as a cashier at a supermarket for almost a year. Besides, there was no room for Mary in any of the units for lower-functioning patients.

Strangely, Mary was calm at meals, a common time for conflicts between other patients. Even when going to meals meant a walk outside, she seemed to know that this was not a "walk," but a meal, and went along quietly, if mechanically. She ate mechanically, too, looking only at her food, ignoring those around her.

A few of the patients had tried making friends with her, but Mary did not respond, and the other patients soon began to avoid her. She became a nonperson in the unit to all but Wendy and Doc. Doc felt challenged and tried at least once a week to break through, to get some kind of engagement from the young woman. He tried in vain. When he asked questions during their sessions, she looked at him wide-eyed and still, and he believed she could be looking through him.

Or she looked away. Once she started crying and Doc thought he had finally made some kind of contact. But when he asked the same questions to start things off the next session, Mary just stared at him.

Wendy never gave up. She didn't know what questions to ask, or what she might do if Mary Johnson answered them, but she knew what patients liked, and she tried her best to give it to them. Most afternoons, Wendy would take Mary back into the dormitory and read her a story from a children's book she borrowed from the library. Mary was always stone silent and still during these stories. Never a laugh or a tear or anything. The most that ever happened— and it happened frequently—was that Mary would go to sleep. She would be awake until the very last page, and then her breathing would even out and she would slump against Wendy's shoulder as the last words of the story were being spoken.

Wendy didn't like to put Mary Johnson into the seclusion room. The room was not uncomfortable in any way. It was a small bed-room furnished with only a single bed. Although in some other units the bed did not have sheets or blankets, this precaution was not believed necessary in Wilson Cottage. The Wilson Cottage beds did not have built-in restraints, either. The seclusion rooms were painted the same dull pastels as the rest of the hospital, and the only windows were the foot-square viewing windows in the doors. The doors locked only from the outside. The rooms, of course, were not supposed to have electrical outlets, but only about half the rooms had been designed as seclusion rooms, so the plugs and light switches had to be removed from the others. The overhead light was well out of reach and the light switch was mounted outside the room.

Mary did not like seclusion. Not many patients did. In most cases, the threat of seclusion was usually enough to help control assaultive behavior. A patient learned that certain acts resulted in seclusion. Naturally, assaultive behavior did not stop completely. Many of the patients had poor control over their impulses, and minor skir-mishes took place fairly regularly.

Most patients, though they didn't like it, just settled down on the mattress and fell asleep once they were put in seclusion. Some tried their best to do damage to the room, picking at the plastic base-board, biting or picking holes in the mattress, tearing apart the sheets. If a patient was known to be suicidal, he or she was either put in restraints, tied to the bed with leather straps, or, if staffing allowed, accompanied in seclusion by a psych tech.

Mary Johnson had not displayed any suicidal behavior. Nor had she attempted to damage the seclusion room, even though she found herself in there at least four or five times a week.

But Mary did not endure seclusion quietly. Perhaps she feared this was just a way station on the trip back to her neighborhood and that the boys who made her take her clothes off would soon be coming for her. Perhaps the room only reminded her of the prison her room at home had become, focusing inward the terror of everything waiting to assault her the moment she stepped outside.

Whatever the reason, within minutes of being left in the seclusion room, Mary would commence slapping her hands on the door. After several minutes of this she would slap harder, and then clench her hands into tight little fists and strike even harder.

The first time Mary did this, the staff responded by opening the seclusion room door. Mary cowered in the far corner of the room immediately. The staff member scolded her, "If you do that, you'll only have to stay in longer."

Within a minute after the staff member closed the door, the pounding would begin again. The staff member would return. Mary would cower again. The staff member would scold her again, close the door, and return to the dayroom or the nursing station. The pounding would begin again.

The seclusion rooms in Wilson Cottage were located on the short hall leading to the bathrooms. The noise from Mary Johnson's pounding was an annoyance not because of the volume, which could be easily masked with a radio, but because it was a form of communication, just about the only time Mary communicated with anyone. Mary was saying something, something more than "Let me out of here," and the inability of anyone to answer her was why the staff's response was, eventually, to ignore the pounding. At first, they would still respond the first three or four times. But soon they responded only twice, then once, then not at all.

Mary's pounding while in seclusion had become a fixture in Wilson Cottage. Some of the staff believed they would eventually find the right combination or dosage of medications to calm her, to dispel her terror and perhaps allow some communication, some therapy, some improvement—to allow Mary to talk to them and they to her. Others figured maybe a bed in one of the back wards would open up and Mary would be somebody else's problem.

One afternoon, when neither Wendy nor Doc was present, Mary clawed one of the other patients, not seriously, but enough to warrant an hour in seclusion. As usual, she did not resist the psych tech who gently but firmly took her by the arm and led her to the room. Within a minute after the door was closed, the pounding began. Since most of the patients were at their jobs, the staff was taking advantage of the time to work on some group therapy with a few of the remaining patients, including Lily Speere. The pounding was a nuisance, but, as before, they were soon able to ignore it and go on with therapy.

Meanwhile, in the seclusion room, Mary had progressed from slaps to clenched fists when she spotted the clean white sheets on the bed. They must have been the same kind of sheets her father and uncle tied her up in before they started climbing all over her and hurting her and making her ashamed. Mary Johnson's eyes glared at the sheets as if they were somehow guilty, as if the sheets themselves were responsible for her pain and they might leap out from the bed all by themselves and wrap themselves around her, and then the bad things would happen. Mary's terror and anger grew together, one nourishing the other. She reached out to the sheets. They were cool and crisp on the skin of her shoulders and neck, and they wrapped so easily, as if they had the same filthy life in them that she had, the same dark looseness of flesh, the same hunger for shame.

She wrapped and wrapped and pulled and pulled and lay down on the floor and rolled against the tension of the sheet still attached under the mattress, and she tugged harder and wrapped tighter. The heat of her skin became the heat of the sheets. The white cloth became soaked with her sweat and yellow on the edges where it pressed into her skin.

Mary felt the shame, then, and the hurt. Her uncle used to grab her neck, so now Mary grabbed her own neck and then pulled on the sheets even tighter and rolled herself up close to the bed and then threw herself back with the full force of her body. The sheet pulled so tight that Mary's mouth opened to gag for air, but there was no sound.

Mary tried to push air out her mouth, but there was no air in her. She clawed at the sheets around her neck, but her own sweat had soaked the cloth and her panicked fingers could not find where the cloth ended and her skin began. Her head began to reel and ache, and she rolled herself around and started pounding on the door.

The first time the pounding had stopped, the staff had hardly noticed. Mary usually pounded the door for the entire hour without stopping, but they were so successful at ignoring it that their subconscious knowledge of the unexpected silence became a deadly partner with their determination to not hear the infernal noise. So although the second pounding was louder and more insistent than the first and all the others before it, no one understood the communication Mary Johnson was trying to make. And when the second silence came, it was almost ten minutes before anyone recognized it as real silence, and decided someone ought to check on Mary Johnson.

They tried to revive her, but the sheets were so tight around her neck that they had to cut them off. No amount of oxygen or CPR or fretting or sliding of blame off the skin like so much sweat could revive her. After her body was removed and the room cleaned up, and the patients who saw the whole thing calmed down—they had to give Lily Speere a tranquilizer to stop her screaming—all anyone could think about was facing Wendy's wrath and Doc's silent disappointment.

22 _____

There were mornings Wendy liked to sit in her truck before going into Wilson Cottage and, like a person settling accounts before a dangerous surgery, collect her worries in front of her and, if not deal them out of her life, at least force them to march in front of her. In the wake of Mary Johnson's suicide, she needed one of these mornings.

Wendy took a deep breath and let the field clear. She heard footsteps crunching the gravel behind her and hoped it wasn't someone who would recognize her and get her out of her truck and into the swing of work before she had a chance to finish her revery. No, it was someone from another unit, who just walked by to his car.

Doc wasn't in a good mood, and Wendy couldn't blame him. He was worried about Greta Lampson. Doc had gone to court and made his case for electroshock therapy, but it was no go. He came back from court about as visibly upset as he ever got. "The woman is suicidal! She is determined to die!" he had said. "And I know this is the only thing that will save her!" But the judge took the advice of

Greta's attorney, who brought in a psychologist who testified that electroconvulsive therapy was a throwback to medieval torture and that Greta's depression would eventually yield to psychotherapy and modern antidepressants.

Doc had shaken his head, muttering "No it won't," and did it again after the judge refused permission for ECT, and did it all the way out of the courtroom.

Doc would come out of it, just as he would come out of his anguish over the death of Mary Johnson. Part of Wendy's admiration for Doc was the way he cared so passionately, but when there was nothing more he could do, when a patient died or left the hospital, Doc felt the pain, and got over it and was right back at the front lines again without missing a step.

Wendy looked at her watch. She had ten minutes left.

Dr. Steven Rose. Wendy couldn't understand why Rosey should be one of her problems. Maybe it was her motherly feelings about the unit, not about the resident. After all, he was messing things up on the unit, as well as letting himself in for major trouble down the line somewhere. If he wanted to fraternize with the patients, fine. Who cares if it destroyed his effectiveness as a psychiatrist, like Doc constantly warned him it would? Who cares if he spent way too much time with Ethel Flynn? Well, Doc cared. Let Doc worry about it, then, as long as Ethel didn't start acting uppity around the unit.

Well fruck-a-duck! Let Doc worry about that, too!

And let Doc worry about how much medication Lily Speere got. Doc had reversed himself and managed to talk the rest of the treatment team into lowering her dose, despite Wendy's protest that the girl was still just lying low. There would be trouble with this one, Wendy felt. Lily displayed a vulnerability that made her seem a lost little girl. She didn't talk much, and when she did, she stammered. A bad sign, in Wendy's view. Lily was still terribly bewildered.

Wendy decided to let Doc worry about that, too. She had learned that there were some things that she just had to let Doc worry about, things that really weren't her responsibility.

There seemed to be more and more of those things, lately. The nurses were taking over a lot of the tasks that had traditionally been handled by psych techs. Wendy couldn't understand it at all. There was a shortage of nurses nationwide. The hospital was strapped for money. And here they were, breaking their backs to hire more and more nurses, mainly to perform jobs that psych techs had been doing for less pay.

Maybe, like Doc said, it was just history. But it was crazy history, and crazy bad luck, as far as Wendy was concerned. So what if the hospitals were becoming more medically oriented. Wendy didn't see them rushing to put more doctors in charge of things, so why should the psych techs get the short end?

Maybe Doc was right, Wendy should just get herself to nursing school.

This was a good problem to let march across her mind as Wendy got out of the truck and headed into Wilson Cottage.

Wendy's keys jingled loudly as she lifted them to the outer door to Wilson Cottage. It was an open unit, but this door was always kept locked during the night and early morning.

Wendy entered and, as expected, found the unit quiet and almost dark. The night staff usually let her be the villain who woke everybody up. Wendy didn't mind, she kind of enjoyed acting like a mother getting her brood out of bed so they wouldn't be late for school.

The office was empty, which Wendy thought was weird. And there was no note in sight.

Maybe they had to take a patient to the infirmary.

Wendy switched on the lights in the office, and then headed for the locked switches in the hall just outside the dayroom.

The first blow fell as she lifted her keys to the switch. Wendy heard a loud twang as her ear was battered. She screamed and shot her arms out reflexively, then whirled, but her attacker was kicking her under her defenses.

Wendy reached for her keys, which were stuck in the switch, but an arm crashed into her breast and she doubled over. Then she felt the fingernails digging in her neck making their way for her face.

Gotta protect my eyes, Wendy thought, and she twisted away violently and crouched down as she covered her head with her arms and tried to bury her face in her chest. She kicked at her attacker and screamed for help.

Now her attacker was climbing on her back, throttling her and reaching around to get a grip on her face. Wendy fell to the floor and tried to roll over on top, or just get away. When she hit the ground her attacker screamed.

Okay, it was a woman. Wendy flapped her elbows out, trying to keep her hands on her eyes. Feeling no contact, she chanced a glimpse.

Zelda Glover's eyes burned with hatred as she reached for Wendy's face.

Wendy screamed and swung a punch at Zelda. Then she remembered that the safest thing, unless her attacker had a knife or some other kind of weapon, was to tackle her around the middle and try to hold her down. Wendy dove for Zelda, screaming, "Help me! Help me!" and wondering where everybody was, and then thinking that Zelda was remarkably nimble to be able to claw her neck in this position.

Wendy pushed Zelda across the floor and into the wall. The other woman grunted, screamed, "Fuck you!" and started kicking and beating at Wendy's head, trying to push her over on to her back. Wendy kept her pinned by pushing with all her might on the slippery floor.

Wendy thought she heard footsteps, but then she felt a warm salty taste in her mouth and her neck felt wet and she tried to remember if Zelda had been tested for the AIDS virus, but couldn't. She thought that was a strange thought to have at the moment when she was fighting for her life.

Then, suddenly, Wendy felt other hands on her, and heard Zelda grunting and groaning. "The bitch attacked me! She hit me!" Zelda sobbed. "I'm hurt, take me to the infirmary!"

Wendy just lay there. Two patients, Henry Dove and Tom Coolidge, another bipolar patient, were holding Zelda back. Bennett Ackerman was standing there like a little boy whose mother had slipped on his banana peel. "Are you okay, Wendy?" he asked.

23 _____

George Konopski took a momentary break from his duties in the V-unit to rub his eyes hard and admit to himself that he no longer felt safe. The boundaries between madness and sanity were no longer holding. Of course, he acknowledged, if those lines held too well, he'd be out of a job.

Konopski sighed and inspected his catalog of woes. He began with the weather. What it was doing outside had gone beyond rain an hour and a half ago. It was a monsoon. Water was pelting the building so hard you could hear it through the walls. Luckily, the V-units were built on high ground. He'd heard that four wards in the hospital had to be evacuated because of flooding.

Konopski's job search at the convention had been a waste of time. George had just been wandering through the exhibit hall when he found himself standing in front of the placement service. The young woman behind the counter caught his eye and he said, "What the hell" to himself and sat down to a huge notebook filled with job listings. There were plenty of jobs, and in some interesting places, too. But Konopski found he had no taste for it. He mechanically flipped through a few more pages, then left.

So here he was, at Bedloe to stay, for better or worse. Mostly worse.

Well, that wasn't exactly true, Konopski admitted to himself, trying to be as rational as he could. He liked his work here. It was a pretty grim place, for sure, but it was exciting psychiatry, and the paychecks came in regularly.

The unit was in good shape. Konopski had a good team assembled here. They kept things clean.

Ned Salmon, poor little guy, would be leaving the unit. Despite Ned's own desire to stay in the hospital, not to mention Konopski's and Alex Greco's medical opinions, the public defender's office had sued for Ned's release and won. So Ned was going to be discharged "AMA," against medical advice.

He had cried when Konopski told him the judge's decision. "There's nothing I can do, Ned," Konopski had said. "You'll be okay, guy."

Hey, Konopski thought, maybe he would be. Maybe the judge and the public defender's office did know better than Ned and his doctors.

Frank Robbins poked his shaved head into the office, "You sign those papers, yet?"

"Oh, not yet. I'll have them in a little bit, Frank," Konopski said without looking at the nurse.

Robbins didn't leave.

"You giving me the once over?"

"You okay?"

Konopski took a deep breath and slammed his hand on the desk. "Yeah, I'm fine. I guess I got up out of the wrong bed this morning. Or got into the wrong car. Or drove to the wrong job."

"Place gets to you, I know," Robbins nodded.

Konopski turned toward the nurse and Robbins noticed his eyes were bloodshot. "Come in. Close the door."

When the door was shut, Konopski motioned Robbins to sit down. "I'll tell you what gets to me. You were here this morning. Did you see our star patient and his guest?"

"Dillinger had a guest? I didn't know. I was here, but I was involved with Ned and some of the other guys."

"I'll tell you what it is."

"His lawyer show up to complain again?"

"Hell, no," Konopski said. "That guy's not going to complain. He's so happy he's got his client in here. He just shows up to let us know he's thinking of us—and to bill the state for a few thousand dollars a shot."

"So who came for Dillinger?"

"His writer girlfriend."

Robbins smiled. "Oh, her. Sure. Conjugal visit?"

"Don't laugh. It'll come to that. It'll come to that." Konopski became more animated now, and tapped Robbins's arm. "Look, she walks in here like the Queen of Sheba, I swear, and announces that she wants to have a visit with Linus Dillinger. And they must have privacy, she says. And then she shows me the letters back and forth and all that stuff. So I tell her privacy might be a problem, but we'll do what we can. I sent them out into the courtyard. There's no way in or out except through the locked double door to this unit. The rain let up temporarily, so what the hell.

"So there they are, out in the courtyard, and I take a look out every now and then, you know, to make sure he's not climbing over the walls or something. And they're just walking up and down the path under the trees, as nice as can be, talking. And then I look again, you know by now they've been out there for almost an hour. And they're holding hands! Just as cute as can be. And I'm seeing the light of love in her eyes. Frank—this guy blew the heads off seven women her age!"

"Well . . . you know . . . there's no accounting for taste. Some women like their men rough."

"She came to the right place, lemme tell you!"

"Well . . . the state wants him outta here. You know that."

"I'd love to see it. I really would."

"But you won't sign the papers."

Konopski closed his eyes and shook his head. "No way. Those bastards'll come after me. He'll have my head rolling on the floor. Only it won't be his shotgun, it'll be his lawyers."

"Akbar wants you to do it," Robbins said.

"Akbar's putting the screws to me. He wants me to do it."

"What are you gonna do?"

"I think I'm gonna get outta town. I—"

Just then there was a crash, shouts, and screams from the enclosed room. Robbins was on his feet and out the door in a flash. Konopski saw a man's body fly through the air and crash into a wall. There was a smear of blood on the glass.

"Call for help," Robbins said. "It's Tang."

Tang was crouched in a martial-arts stance in the far corner. There was blood on his wrists, either from hitting another man, or perhaps from slipping out of the leather straps, Konopski thought. Jesse and Rocco were already in the room, coming between Tang and the other patients, most of whom were cowering along the walls, covering their heads or crawling away. A few, though, were approaching Tang, clenching their fists.

"Get a riot crew down here right away!" Konopski shouted into the phone, then hung up and dashed out to follow Robbins into the dayroom.

"Stand back, Doc!" Robbins cautioned below his voice. "I think I can take him."

"Oh no you can't, Frank. Just leave him be until the crew gets here. Leave him be!"

One of the patients who had been posturing in front of Tang suddenly took a step forward and the Asian moved upon him in a blur that sent the other man flying backward, blood streaming from his nose. Tang danced toward the other men who were still standing and, in another blur, beat them back, doubled up and bloody.

Robbins moved forward, palms flattened out in front of him. "Easy there, Tang. Easy there."

Tang, back in his corner, crouched down, and his eyes became dry black holes. Robbins took a slow step forward while Jesse and Rocco and Konopski ushered and dragged the other patients out of the room.

"Get the gook!" one of the other patients yelled. Some of the men were crying. Some were cursing.

Tang screamed and kicked a chair, leaving one wooden leg in splinters.

"Easy, Tang. Easy!" Robbins took another step forward.

"Wait for the team, Frank!" Konopski shouted.

"Hey, Tang, I thought we were buddies." Robbins took another step closer to Tang.

The buzzer rang and the riot team let themselves in with their own key.

"The team's here, Frank. Hold on."

"Shit, I trained that team!" Robbins muttered as he took another step toward Tang. He was only about two yards away.

Tang picked up a chair, whirled, and threw it crashing through the plate-glass window. Robbins ducked and went in toward Tang's waist.

Tang danced under the much larger man's grip, shifted the weight of both, and spun Robbins over and down, delivering a kick to his midsection and then his face. He stood over Robbins and was about to kick his head when three men from the team jumped on his back. He screamed and rolled over, carrying the three with him. Robbins came to and backed away. One of the men came flying toward him. The other two were being punched and kicked by the screaming blur Tang had become.

"Get outta there!" Konopski cried out.

Robbins dragged one man out, and the other two slipped around and escaped. Tang danced across to the other side of the room, smashing chairs on his way.

"Doctor Konopski, do you have a shot ready or should we use ours?" one of the team members asked, referring to a tranquilizer.

"Son, this is one place where we've always got a shot ready. But I don't think Mr. Tang is ready for his shot quite yet. At least he doesn't think so."

"We'll hold him down. You tranquilize him."

"You and what army? You've been here the last couple minutes, haven't you?"

"Get that shot ready."

The man, a thin, wiry psych tech Konopski had never seen before, pulled a backpack off his shoulder and opened it. He pulled out a package and started unwrapping it.

"A net?" Konopski muttered.

"A net," Jesse repeated.

"C'mere, Frank," the man said to Robbins, who was holding a towel to his nose. "You know how to do this, right?"

"I showed you how to do it, remember?"

"Oh, right. Well, let's go. Jack. Fred! Jesse. Rocco. Doctor."

"Get behind us, Doctor Konopski, " Frank said as the six of them took slow, careful steps into the room and then approached Tang, whose eyes glared at them. He muttered something the men couldn't understand.

"That sounded like one hell of a curse," Robbins said.

"I think he was just welcoming us back for another round," Jesse said.

"You're all wrong," Konopski said. "He was thinking out loud that we're the ones who're crazy, for coming in after him again."

When they were three yards away Tang tensed.

"He's moving again," Rocco whispered.

"Hike!" Robbins yelled. The men threw the net over Tang, who screamed and started whirling and kicking. But the more he whirled and kicked and punched the tighter the net wound around him.

"Now yank it!" Robbins said.

Tang was now a mummy twisting in the cocoon, and the men were upon him.

"Get the legs, Jesse! Rocco, help the doctor."

As Konopski approached, hypodermic preloaded with a powerful tranquilizer, the little man started to cry.

24

Konopski was not surprised when he got the call from Alex. There was not much else that could have gone screwy. His prayers for an end to the rain had been answered. With a vengeance. The monsoons of the previous month had abruptly ceased, and the skies cleared. Now it hadn't rained for weeks and the politicians were threatening to ration water. Just about all of Konopski's neighbors had stopped watering their lawns. He didn't mind letting the grass die, but he was not about to see his tomato plants shrivel. So he snuck out every night at eleven and watered them.

And whoever said dry heat was better than humid heat never spent much time inside Bedloe State Hospital when it was ninety dry degrees. Your sweat dried so damn fast that all the fans brought in by staff members from home only blew the air around inside the oven.

The news about Ned Salmon, who had been released almost a month ago, was not good. But it wasn't the worst news Konopski received that day. That came in person from Sam Akbar, the Superintendent-Almighty himself. Akbar had summoned George to his office and said he was going to make the whole Linus Dillinger matter very simple. Then he proceeded to "require" that Konopski perform a psychiatric evaluation on the patient within the next two weeks.

Konopski had an answer all ready, though he had to fight the choke back down his throat in order to deliver it. His good friend and attorney, Allan DiMara, had advised him to "avoid the thing" as long as possible. "Just don't do it. Put it off. Don't have the time, that's all. You're a busy doctor."

But the avoiding was all done now. The requests, official and otherwise, the cajoling, the almost-friendly threatening were all done. Akbar had made it clear that this was going to be a formal request, made in writing, acknowledging past requests and memos on the subject.

"I just wanted to give you a chance to avoid all that and get it done."

Konopski was ready, thanks to Allan, with one more card to play.

"Well," he had said to Akbar, "I'll do it, but it's got to be by the book."

Akbar had raised his eyebrows. "What do you mean?"

Konopski cleared his throat. "I want my attorney present, I want the attorney general present, I want Dillinger's attorney present, and I want the whole thing recorded by the court."

"What the hell are you trying to do?"

"That's what I want, that's all. That's by the book."

Konopski hoped Akbar didn't ask him which book. The whole idea was Allan DiMara's. George had heard of attorneys being present during forensic psychiatric evaluations before, but it wasn't exactly routine. And he'd never heard of the prosecutor being there. In fact, it was probably illegal.

Akbar took a deep breath, shuffled some papers around the top of his desk, and said he'd see what he could do.

After awhile, when Konopski had calmed down, he realized that he might have played his hand a little too soon. After all, Akbar had said the formal request hadn't been prepared yet.

Well, so what? Konopski thought, so this was just another threat. He probably could have bought more time by just doing nothing. Well, so what? Anything more, I'll let DiMara handle it, that's all, he decided.

So when Alex Greco called with the news about Ned Salmon,

Konopski was not prepared to be amazed or particularly disappointed in the way the universe took care of things.

Salmon had thrown a brick through a shop window. "That's our Ned," Konopski had said. Konopski could almost have predicted it. Salmon wasn't prepared for the outside world. He had been practically born and raised in mental hospitals. Now, both to Ned's doctors and to the public defender's office, this was a horrible tragedy. But where the public defender's office saw the solution in getting Ned out of the hospital and keeping him out, Ned's psychiatrists saw Ned as a human being who would never be able to live outside a setting as highly structured as a hospital.

The report—which Alex had received through unofficial channels because as far as the law was concerned Ned was a private citizen now and his connection with Bedloe was terminated—said that Ned had not shown up for his last two appointments at the community mental health center where he was supposed to report once a week to receive his medications, and that he had not been seen around his single-room-occupancy hotel for five days.

Konopski knew Salmon had not thrown the brick in anger, it was more likely frustration, or just a boilover from his witch's brew of a mind. Ned would never hurt anyone or anything on purpose. Ned did hardly anything on purpose.

"Well, so I suppose we'll be seeing our little friend again soon," Konopski had remarked.

"No. The judge let him go," Alex said.

"What?"

"Gave him another chance. Apparently the psychologist for the community mental health center pleaded brilliantly on his behalf."

"More likely on his budget's behalf," Konopski spat. "Jesus!" Because Ned was a penal code patient, one who had committed crimes, there was more money readily available for whatever facility was at the moment responsible for his care. And code patients like Ned were a prize: easy to manage and not really dangerous. Most of the time they hardly ever showed up. But the checks kept coming on time. So Ned was worth fighting for, and the community mental health center had fought for him, and won.

"Christ! They didn't even call us in!" Konopski gasped. "The poor bastard!"

"The judge decided to give him another chance," Alex said.

"To do what?"

25

The little man felt the ripe quality of the air spreading out before him. He had no knowledge of how far the air kept going beyond his fingertips, which were now reaching out in front of him, riding the billowing dark wind.

He could see the ground more than a hundred feet straight below his perch in the administration tower. If he directed his eyes on an angle away from the tower, the ground became farther and farther away, until it disappeared in the black horizon.

He had no knowledge of his name. Tang was a word that was thrown at him, but the word had no roots in his heart. He had no knowledge of his heart. It disappeared somewhere inside him beyond some black edge.

For someone with his training, escape from the ward was not difficult. He had no knowledge of his training, though his muscles and that part of his mind which controlled them were still quick and clever.

He smelled rain in the air, and this made his chest flutter. He did not know why, but the sweet damp smell in the air was pushing some massive hurt up into his head, something loathsome and terrible. The wind came down past him and swept leaves and birds out of a huge tree below.

He registered the distance and direction of sounds that reached him from below: voices, car doors, footsteps, laughter. The cleverness that was still alive in his mind knew he was safe here, no one below could see him.

Clouds moved and the moon lit up the world spread out before him. There was a sudden light on the horizon, and then it went dark again. He had no knowledge of what it could have been, but he stared at the place where the light had been.

The air quickened. This time it was not a gust, there was half a world behind it. From his shelter in the tower, he sensed the increasing strength of the wind from the way it rushed past and called him with its soothing, whispered wail. There was a series of sudden explosions of light behind him. His eyes widened and the cleverness in his mine was alerted. The world rumbled. His muscles tensed. When the wind brought the last humid flush pregnant with rain, he felt it and knew what it was, knew what would be coming just behind it. He could hear the armies coming, needles racing along the earth.

He leapt, and as he felt the wind caress him and carry him toward the horizon, the knowledge of sorrow and anguish ripped through him and flew from his mouth as he cried the names of his wife and children.

26

Firing Dean Lester was only the first step in cleaning up D-7. Lester had been the director of the ward, which meant the person Alex hired to replace him would have more authority than if Lester had been merely the physician assigned to the unit. But Alex had to move fast. He went through the motions of putting ads in several newspapers and psychiatric journals, but then made a telephone call.

More than a decade ago, Veronica Uyemura had been one of Alex's best psychiatric residents at a hospital on the West Coast. The woman had the straight backbone, forthright attention to detail, and too-sure-to-be-denied voice of a drill sergeant. Alex was in luck: Dr. Uyemura was currently in one of those slumps many good psychiatrists find themselves in at certain times in their careers. She was working as a psych-temp and was more than ready to say yes to his request. Alex refused to hire her until she inspected the hospital. "I don't want you to get into something on the strength of my recommendation and then find out you made a mistake."

Uyemura was only a few minutes into her tour of D-7 when she told Alex she'd seen enough and asked him to come outside with her. When she was sure they could not be overheard, she said, "Alex, that unit is positively medieval. What worries me about coming here is how you could allow that to exist in your hospital."

All Alex said was, "Will you come, Ronnie?"

"Will I be able to change anything? I won't preside over this."

"You'll be able to put the unit in good medical trim."

"I've heard that before, Alex. That psych tech, Penny Scott. I've seen burnout, but that woman is a sadist."

Alex took a deep breath and nodded. "We'll have trouble with the union, but she'll go. Does that mean you'll take the job?"

"I want to hire my own staff. Everyone in that hellhole goes. Everyone."

Walking to his car, she stopped in the shade of a beech tree and turned back to look at the hospital. "How could I refuse this chance? It will be like going back in time one hundred, maybe two hundred or more years—carrying with me the tools of modern psychiatry to this place!"

Uyemura's first responsibility was to see to the medical needs of the patients. Within a few hours of her arrival, she began sending patients to the hospital infirmary. A few had to be sent to Valley Hospital, not only because some of their medical problems were too severe to be treated at Bedloe, but also because the infirmary was already swamped with patients from D-7.

Uyemura wanted a completely new staff, and Alex did his best to give it to her. He reviewed the records of all the D-7 staff, then called in the officers of the respective unions. He showed them the evidence, which consisted of photographs, complaints by relatives of patients, medical records from the Bedloe infirmary and Valley Hospital, and reports filed by Doc and Dr. Uyemura. He declared, that on the basis of the shameful conditions in the unit, he could dismiss everyone connected with it, as he had already done with Dean Lester.

But Alex said he didn't believe that was necessary. What he proposed was this: Staff who had appeared to perform well before they got to D-7 would be transferred to other units. Staff members with spotty prior records would be put on probation and transferred to less critical duties, or fired. After an hour or so of blustering and posturing, the union officers agreed to Alex's terms. Since Dr. Uyemura had already been recruiting the staff she wanted, within a few days, D-7 had a completely new crew: psychologist Dan Billings, psychiatric social worker Timothy Buck, half a dozen new psych techs, rehabilitation therapist Faith Dundee, and something D-7 never had before—a music therapist, by the name of Dolores Woods.

Alex received plenty of threatening phone calls during July, all anonymous. He thought of having his number changed, but when he called his former mother-in-law to tell her to notify Carmen of the impending change, she said she had no idea where Alex's daughter was. So the change was canceled and Alex and his family endured the calls until they trailed off in early August.

[2]

Veronica Uyemura was a crackerjack psychiatrist and she had assembled a formidable team. But she knew the problems of D-7 could overwhelm the best staff. She was grateful that while her new staff came on most of the patients were out of the unit, in the infirmary or Valley Hospital. The next order of business was to review the medications of every patient in D-7. Some were getting too much of the wrong drugs, some not enough of the right ones. She knew that until they were able to get their symptoms under greater control, trying to accomplish anything else would be futile. She took the patient files home to have more time to review them, and called the treatment teams together on a crisis basis. Within two weeks they had overhauled the medication programs of every patient in D-7.

Early on in the process, Uyemura had come to Alex especially to talk about a few of her new patients, including Walter Channing.

"He's a good boy, but he's so ill, and he's not responding to standard antipsychotic medications. I want to try lithium," she said.

That was Uyemura. Right to the point. Lithium was not traditionally used for schizophrenia but was standard in the treatment of bipolar disorder, or manic-depression. But there had been some reports of success with lithium in schizophrenia, and Uyemura wanted to try it.

"Some of his early diagnoses were for bipolar disorder," she pointed out.

"And at least one schizoaffective, too," Alex said.

Uyemura smiled. "I'm glad some things haven't changed. You still know the files of all your patients."

Alex was silent. Then he said, "You're the doctor."

"Don't try that on me. I want to know what you think."

"I think you're the doctor."

"Alex, really, Doctor."

Alex sighed. "He's a tough case. Nothing else has worked. Go ahead."

[3]

To Alex, social worker Timothy Buck appeared somewhat thin around the edges, and maybe a bit too light for the winds that could blow around Bedloe. Uyemura characterized her second-in-command in the unit as a sensitive and capable professional who cared about patients.

Timothy Buck walked into the unit his first day, dropped the piles of paperwork that were required of him, cast a slow, steady glance around and pronounced, "Nobody's having any fun in here!" He then proceeded to get every patient left in the unit dressed and out the door for a walk around the grounds. On that walk, which was supported by two new psych techs and the rehabilitation therapist, Buck abruptly stopped when they came over a hill.

"What's that? It looks like a farm," Buck said, pointing at a small, flat valley in the southeastern corner of the grounds.

It was a farm, or had been one. Timothy Buck, who had grown up on a farm in Iowa, decided it would be a farm again.

Bedloe State Hospital was conceived and built during a period when care for the mentally ill was patterned on the concept of asylum. There were potions, concoctions, and various mechanical therapies to be administered, of course, but they did little good. At least, they did not do enough good to allow very many of the mentally ill to lead normal lives in society. So hospitals were designed to be places of refuge, providing not only a place to live but also activities to occupy mind and body. Within their walls, state hospitals were models of small towns, with their own municipal services and responsibilities, their own electrical power plants and water departments, their own blacksmiths and mechanical shops, their own bakeries, fire and police departments, post offices, libraries, barbershops, beauty parlors, and farms.

Patients took on whatever responsibilities their level of functioning allowed. The medical assumption was that honest work was therapeutic, and the assumption was correct. The best hospitals buzzed with productivity behind walls that protected their patients from the violence and stress of everyday life in society.

Naturally, the concept of asylum was not always represented at its best. Many hospitals became little more than human chicken coops, and even those that made an honest attempt at asylum fell victim to the general notion that in order to appear worthy of its public trust and financing, a hospital had to demonstrate effectiveness in "curing" mental illness. They accomplished this by discharging patients at regular intervals. Whether the patient was ready to leave the hospital or not was another matter. Most were not, but the revolving doors installed in mental hospitals served the purposes of the bureaucracy: hospital administrators could point to their high discharge rates and claim effective treatment, and then point to the high admissions rate and claim their institutions were serving a dire need.

Bedloe had been among the grandest and most ambitious state hospitals in design, an almost totally self-sufficient physical plant able to support a community of over twenty thousand patients and staff. The apple, pear, and peach orchard alone covered more than ten acres. The flat, miniature valley in the southeastern corner of the grounds had once contained more than five acres of vegetables: tomatoes, beans, lettuce, potatoes, turnips, beets, and squash.

All that was left of this cornucopia were many faded black-and-white photographs of patients smiling as they embraced their champion pumpkins and monster turnips. There were different reasons why the farm fell into disuse. According to stories Alex heard from Wendy Dixon, and which he confirmed while sifting through some dusty file cabinets, the farm had been in almost full operation right up to around 1972. The deinstitutionalization war of attrition had drained not only resources but also spirit from the hospital. The optimists among the staff saw themselves as caretakers who were phasing out an obsolete institution, but most of the staff were not optimistic. Why plant seeds and tend young trees on a farm that was to be abandoned?

Labor unions and civil liberties suits dealt the final blow to the farm by demanding that the patients receive standard wages for their work. The hospital could not afford it, so the farm was shut down.

Alex had not blackened his hands searching for records on Bedloe's farm just to satisfy his curiosity. He was gathering ammunition. At Veronica Uyemura's urging and on the strength of Wendy's hunch, Alex found himself in the dank basement of the administration building sifting through files covered with the oily black dust of two decades. Buck had convinced Uyemura that working the Bedloe farm would be "a terrific way to get the patients outside, doing something productive—and there's enough summer left for a quick crop, too." Uyemura had taken the request to Alex.

He had frowned. "That's not a medical thing. I know Akbar's going to have a hard time with it. It'll cost money."

"Not that much," Uyemura said. "The tractors are still in use—they mow the lawns with them. And the rest of the necessary equipment is in the farm shed. We checked."

Alex knew that the relative cost was not the issue, and Uyemura knew that, too. Institutions don't cease fulfilling their mission because of thriftiness, however misguided, but because of inertia. They would need more than working tractors to budge Akbar.

"I have an idea. Let me work on this," Alex said.

"Buck made a copy of the farm shed key," Uyemura said. "He'll work it without permission if he has to. After all, you can't see the farm from the hospital proper. By the time we get caught, we'll be eating salad we grew ourselves."

But Uyemura and Buck and the patients of D-7 did not have to become secret farmers. Alex found what he was looking for in the old files. So when he went to Sam Akbar to talk about reviving the Bedloe farm, he was ready. As expected, Akbar smiled at the idea, said it was great, and then shook his head sorrowfully that it couldn't be done because it was so expensive. Alex knew that arguing that it would cost next to nothing was useless. No matter how many tools and tractors were still around, reviving the farm would cost something, and Akbar was the arbiter of whether any amount was too much.

Unless, of course, it was a medical procedure.

Which, Alex reminded him, it was. In the old files, Wendy's hunch had been confirmed: a physician had been in charge of the Bedloe farm for most of its history, including the last thirty years of its operation. Furthermore, whether or not a patient could or should work on the farm was decided exclusively by physicians. The farm had always been under the supervision of the medical staff, which made it Alex's responsibility.

"It will look good to the accreditation committee," Alex philosophized as he turned and left Sam's office.

So Buck, Uyemura, and the patients of D-7 got their farm.

27 _____

One of the staff members would later reminisce that the renaissance in D-7 began "with people just being nicer." This was no doubt true. But as far as psychiatrist Veronica Uyemura was concerned, the prime ingredient in the rebirth of D-7 as a functioning hospital ward wasn't going to be compassion. It wasn't going to be skill. It was going to be attention. Dr. Uyemura hired people she knew would have no trouble fulfilling her expectation that every staff member would not only give attention to the patients, but pay it as well. This was not only most important, but it could be easily measured in the minutes a staff member spent in proximity or direct interaction with patients.

Veronica Uyemura had walked in and found a unit without leadership, adrift, and she knew that when a human enterprise drifts, it is seldom toward a better haven. She found a unit that was dark until noon, where patients rambled around undressed or in pajamas, hungry. So when she first assembled her new staff, she mandated that the unit would always be fully lit by seven every morning and that patients would be dressed and back from breakfast by 8:30.

Veronica, social worker Timothy Buck, and psychologist Dan Billings knew that the unit needed a lot of rehabilitation before they could get on with the more advanced activities like group supportive therapy meetings. By virtue of the neglect of the old D-7 staff, the unit had deteriorated into something no zookeeper would tolerate, though most governors and state mental health authorities managed to blink at similar or worse conditions quite nicely. Part of what the staff would remember most was that they had found a ward where many patients had lived together for several years, and yet most didn't know any of their fellow patients' names. The patients needed to be brought back into the human race.

To aid in the effort, Uyemura and Timothy Buck had hired Faith Dundee, the rehabilitation and occupational therapist, and Dolores Woods, the music therapist. These were not luxury positions. The idea was not that D-7's patients might someday be holding down jobs on Main Street or filling in for the city philharmonic. But then again, Faith, a short, chubby elf with fiery red hair exploding in curls, and Dolores, a tall thin woman with long black braids, would not have bet against themselves or their patients.

Faith had known she wanted to be a therapist since the ninth grade. Dolores had left a high-paying job on Wall Street to live in a dormitory while a student in training. She claimed no great dedication, however, for her midlife flight from the stock exchange. "I was bored and I wanted to work with some other human emotions besides greed."

Both women knew the minute they walked into the unit that job training and music would have to come a little later. The needs of the patients in D-7 were much more basic. They needed to be taught how to offer a glass of water to another person, how to pour the water into a glass, or how to accept it from another. Many of them needed to be taught how to drink a glass of water.

Faith and Dolores taught them how to find out what day it was, what the weather was like, and what that meant in the scheme of things. They spent a whole week on how to know if someone was dressed right for the weather.

They spent two weeks on the answer to this question: *How are you feeling today?*

They saved for later the lesson on reading from a menu and ordering at a restaurant.

Grooming was a major issue in the new D-7. Many patients had to be taught how to take a shower, how to shave, and how to get dressed. The therapists drew a big list on construction paper of all the major stops on the self-grooming path, and tacked it to the wall near the bathroom. Every patient had his own self-grooming check-list on the sign: *I will get dressed every day. I will wear my shoes every day. I will shave every day. I will keep my shirt clean.*

Some patients had more trouble than others with specific tasks. Most of them had trouble with shoes and socks. Shoes were "borrowed" freely at first and the staff tried to keep some emergency extras on hand. For the first few weeks, they did not require both shoes to be the same, although each had to be on the correct foot. Stealing was sharply reduced when Dolores suggested they institute the "buddy system," in which patients were responsible for helping others.

As each patient successfully completed a grooming task, he checked it off next to his name. When an entire week went by with every task marked off, the unit would be rewarded. At first, the rewards were simple: an extra turn around the ballfield during their morning walk. Faith had bigger things in mind, however: a party to which D-5, the female unit, would be invited.

First, however, the men in D-7 would need to learn how to say hello, begin a conversation, and end one. So Faith and Dolores practiced the art of conversation with them: *Nice day we're having? How are you?*

Naturally, some patients had more trouble with this than others. While Walter Channing, on most days, could be counted on to lead the way in charming conversation, Ralph Webster, a schizophrenic man who had been at Bedloe for twelve years, had his own ideas on what kind of social intercourse he would conduct. Confused as his mind was by his disease, certain of Ralph's other faculties were in excellent shape. He developed an immediate, crushing lust for Dolores Woods. In this passion he was joined by just about every male staff member and a good proportion of the other patients.

Ralph, however, had a unique of method of courtship. When Dolores arrived on the unit in the morning, he stared at her with the steel-eyed concentration of a hawk.

Although it was annoying, everyone in the unit, including the patients, was accustomed to this from Ralph. It was his way of not only beginning a conversation, but it was also his way of conducting and ending one.

Except in the case of Dolores he went several steps further. Ralph had a lot more to say to her.

Dolores usually breezed right past Ralph and into the nursing station for the morning review, in which the staff would discuss the events on the ward during the previous twenty-four hours. It was a mini-treatment-team meeting.

For the first several weeks, Ralph just followed Dolores, stopped short of the door to the nursing station, and continued sending her those silent, unblinking love letters with his eyes. Not wanting to encourage him, Dolores started sitting with her back to the window.

Ralph apparently decided to exercise his passion whatever way he could. One day, in the middle of the meeting, Faith looked up from her notes and immediately grabbed Dolores's knee. "Don't turn around, Dolores, just don't."

Ralph was licking the glass partition separating him from the object of his affection. Other patients were cheering him on as he outlined Dolores's head and neck and shoulders with his tongue and then used it as a painter would a brush to color in a portrait of his love.

Because he wasn't hurting anyone, the staff did not attempt to restrain Ralph, although he was asked to please stop. But the window licking went on for weeks because the man had no other way to express himself.

Well, actually he did, as the staff found out one warm summer morning. The staff has grown accustomed to Ralph and his protestations of love. An extra few bottles of window cleaner were kept handy, and a chair was saved for Dolores so she could keep her back to the window. Suddenly, in the middle of the meeting, Faith grabbed Dolores's knee again.

"I really mean it, Dolores, don't turn around. Really."

Ralph had decided licking the window had brought him all the satisfaction it was going to, so he had escalated his affections.

"What's he doing?" Dolores asked, keeping her body rigid.

Ralph had dropped his pants and was masturbating against the glass.

Faith squeezed Dolores's knee and with the other hand pointed directly at Ralph, got his attention, and said, "Now Ralph, no one appreciates that. So will you please put that thing away now."

There was something in Faith's voice, a quality of determination tempered with kindness that stood her well in these situations. Though his passion for Dolores would never end, Ralph's resolve was deflated. He obeyed Faith and walked away from the window.

To be sure, Faith was better at handling such incidents than Dolores. In fact, these delicate matters were usually left to her by the other staff as well. In the old D-7, where patients wandered around naked or half-dressed most of the time, masturbation was commonly practiced anywhere and everywhere. In the new D-7, where a high premium was put on starting and finishing the day fully dressed, the patients were asked, most often by Faith, to "please go in your bed and do that."

Faith inspired romances of her own. In particular, a little Asian gentleman, Mr. Chen, a patient at Bedloe for a decade, would always smile at her fondly and, every chance he got, offer her a dollar. "Give you a dollah, a dollah!" he would say with the enthusiasm of a prince offering his kingdom.

"What for?" she finally asked him one day.

"Outside, give quarter, can hold lady's hand. Two quarter, get kiss-kiss. Give you a dollah!" he gesticulated.

Faith smiled. "Keep your money," she said, and took his hand in both of hers, for she saw only memories of lechery in the liquid film over the little man's eyes. After that, every now and then she would hold Mr. Chen's hand for a few minutes each day. Once in a while she'd remind him not to go any further than her wrist, and Mr. Chen seemed to appreciate the warning, because when he nodded and smiled, his eyes twinkled.

There was a catatonic patient, silent and frail, who drew Faith's attention during the part of the morning grooming ritual when she handed out clean socks to the men. This man, Leo, sat on his bed and watched as most of the others crowded around to get their socks. Faith always went over to him, handed him his socks, and made sure he was able to get them on. Though she tried to make eye contact, she knew the stony lack of expression on his face was a consequence of his illness and that she should not expect a smile, even in his eyes. She knew Leo spent most of his time standing against a wall somewhere, hands in his pockets.

So when one morning after Faith had been at Bedloe six weeks, Leo walked up to her and said, "Thank you, you're a nice lady," it was a few moments before she could respond in kind.

[2]

Tim Buck's plans for the Bedloe farm were, even he acknowledged, optimistic. With the help of some members of the grounds crew who came in on their own time, an acre was plowed. Tim and the staff recruited some of the higher functioning patients, including Walter Channing, to prepare the plowed ground for planting. After several days of hacking at the earth with rakes and hoes, they did manage to plant some beans and lettuce in one small corner of the acre. The rest of the acre went unused until Faith bought twenty-dollars' worth of wildflower seeds with her own money and organized a planting excursion. Sowing wildflower seeds did not require a level of functioning much beyond being able to walk, hold out one's hand to receive a scoop of seeds, and then fling the seeds onto the ground. Or into the air. Or atop one's head. Or on one's clothes. Or at a fellow patient. Or into one's mouth.

After having been cooped up for the years-long winter of Dean Lester's rule in D-7, most of the patients loved going outdoors. A major portion of the campaign was devoted to outdoor excursions. Tim, Faith, Dolores, and the rest of the staff took the patients on van rides all over the Bedloe Valley. There were hikes and picnics around the grounds as well as in public parks. And Tim and Faith plotted future camping trips at Poe Lake.

Not all of the patients took well to leaving the security of the unit. Several were afraid at first, but soon responded to the cajoling of the staff. Two men flatly refused to leave the unit and would cower and beg piteously. One man would finally leave, but then escape from the group and find his way back to the unit. Another wasn't so fortunate. After being persuaded to leave, he grew more tense as the walk took him further and further from his familiar surroundings. Finally, in a panic, he bolted from the group and into the woods.

Timothy Buck sent the psych techs after the patient and took the others back to the unit on the run. He immediately called the hospital police and instructed them that a penal code patient had escaped and was headed for the woods.

"That man's not a penal code patient," Faith told him. "He's a lamb."

"I know," Tim said.

"Then why did you tell them he's a code?"

"Because I know from experience that if they think he's a code patient they'll pull out all the stops to find him."

Tim had heard the story about the patient who ran off into the woods around Bedloe the previous year. The unit staff was certain he was too ill to find his way to a road and would be wandering around in the hills, and they requested a helicopter and a search party for the large tracts of wilderness above the hospital proper. But because the patient was not a code and so was not considered a danger to the community, only a limited search of the grounds was made. Three days later the man was found by a hunter in the woods, dead from exposure and extreme symptoms of withdrawal from his medications.

This time, however, two helicopters were sent out by the state police to look for the "dangerous escaped lunatic," as the local newspaper reported, who was found later the same afternoon sitting under a tree counting the weeds and ferns he had picked.

[3]

As the renaissance of D-7 continued, the staff realized that as much as they were doing, they weren't doing enough. Timothy Buck and Dan Billings reminded everyone to take encouragement from any and all signs of progress. So they measured their success in the declining use of the seclusion rooms as well as in the rising frequency of smiles. There were fewer and fewer gaps on the daily grooming checklist, and patients made great strides in the art of conversation and other social skills.

When Leo, the catatonic patient, not only secured his own socks and shoes one morning but also approached Faith Dundee and asked her for a date, the staff decided it was time to at least mention the possibility of a party with the women in D-5. This announcement was greeted with applause, some nervous pacing and thrusting of hands into pockets, titters and whispered jokes remembered from high school, and general great cheer.

Timothy Buck decided some of the patients had more than mastered the challenge of ordering from a menu, so he and Dan Billings and a psych tech took ten patients, including Walter Channing, to a local pizza parlor. Studying the menu, Walter began recounting an imaginary menu of all possible pizza combinations. When the waitress came to take his order, she said to him, "You're weird."

Walter looked her straight in the eyes and said, "Yes I am, but not that weird." Then he looked at Dan, smiled, slapped his hand on the table, and asked the waitress if she'd like to dance.

She begged off, on account of her job. Walter, unfazed, asked Dan if it would be all right if he danced by himself. Dan gave him a quarter for the jukebox, but later had to get change for more music when three of the other patients joined Walter.

[4]

Bedloe, like most state hospitals, had a Central Services Department whose job it was to provide equipment and space for various activities. Bedloe's had a music room with a small orchestra's worth of instruments, a graphic arts center, an occupational therapy shop, a small gym, and a photographic lab. Tim and Dan found that these facilities were sorely underutilized, mainly because it was difficult for the patients to get off the wards to use them. They accepted this as a boon for D-7 and began appropriating as much of the equipment as they could.

On their first shopping trip in Central Services, Faith and Dolores found a brand-new video camcorder and immediately signed it out. They could hardly wait to set it up and videotape their social-skills sessions. Most of the patients, though a bit suspicious at first, warmed up considerably once they saw themselves on television. A few were embarrassed and tried to cover the screen with their bodies. One patient denied that it was him on the screen. "That's not me—what are you trying to do to me?"

Although Dolores found a wealth of musical instruments at Central Services, she held off bringing any back to the unit. She felt it would be weeks before the patients were ready for them. In the meantime, she took aside a dozen or so patients at a time for a simple music-therapy session designed to help them express themselves. She began with a simple "hello song," which she would sing to them and then have each patient sing in return. Then each man would sing his name and how he felt. They would close with a "goodbye song." Dolores knew she was making progress when some of the most chronically disabled patients, those who seldom spoke or interacted with anyone, gathered around the nursing station window in the morning upon her arrival and sang the hello song to her. Ralph, her schizophrenic Romeo, was among them.

With new access to athletic equipment, the staff not only introduced stretching and toning sessions, but also played basketball, volleyball, and softball with the patients. Many of the most chronic and socially clumsy patients seemed transformed when they had a ball in their hands. Tim and Dan made careful note of this fact, and checked their calendar to count the days until the hospital's own version of the olympic games. Maybe, they agreed. Just maybe.

Meanwhile, D-7's use of Poe Lake and the hiking trails increased. The first few actual overnight camping trips with a half a dozen patients went fine, so Tim and Dan planned trips with up to a dozen men. More and more patients were enjoying the hikes, including a group of seven very ill, almost completely nonverbal schizophrenic patients Faith would take on two- and three-hour walks in the woods. On one such hike, they came upon an eight-foot-high chain fence. Faith decided to let the patients decide what to do.

For several minutes the seven patients just stood there and looked at the fence. A few touched it, very tentatively. Finally, several minutes later, Andy, a man Faith described as "the most chronic, most nonverbal, most out-of-it patient" decided they should all turn around and go back to find a different trail, which is what they did.

Not all patients improved on all fronts. One man, Rick, was a "screamer." As Faith described him to a psych tech who was filling in one Saturday, "He's so tortured by his hallucinations he just needs release. If something's going on and he gets excited, he doesn't know how to express himself. So he screams. Then he tips over tables or throws chairs. Sometimes he assaults other patients or staff. He can't tolerate loud noises, either. Speak almost in a whisper when you're around him."

Rick was not a favorite in D-7. By September he had assaulted every new staff member and most of the patients. Then, one evening early in the month he started to wail. Before long, his crying was completely out of control. In between the loud sobs, he would try to catch his breath, and choke, and then breathe out a long, wailing sigh. The staff decided to put him in restraints, but no one seemed to be able to look anybody else in the eye while they were doing it.

Afterward, as Rick's suffering drifted on tides no one could measure or control, everyone on the ward withdrew into silence. Patients and staff shared, but did not acknowledge, except by their closed lips and averted eyes, their frustration and their terror. All wanted Rick to be taken care of, sent somewhere he could be fixed or at least separated from them. But there was nowhere to send him. Everyone knew that Rick, and they, were already in that place as far removed as anyone ever got. Rick reminded them all that as much as they were doing, no one could do enough.

28

For the third time one day in early August Alex picked up the document and remembered the first time he had read it, alone at his kitchen table after arriving home near midnight from the Family Organization meeting. Fran had given him a copy at the end of the meeting. Flustered after telling the entire packed church basement about his daughter, Alex had hurried out without even looking at it.

But once he got home, he didn't want to carry his anxious energy to bed, so he sat down with a cup of tea and the report, hoping a little reading might calm him.

Report of the Family Organization Survey: Serious Problems in Patient Care at Bedloe State Hospital. The first page explained that the survey began as a questionnaire summarizing the most common complaints heard at Organization meetings. It promised anonymity and requested information about the personal experiences of the members and their relatives in the hospital. The questionnaire committee was nearly overwhelmed with responses, the introduction said.

Alex turned the page and looked it over quickly, then scanned the next few pages. He closed the book and looked away, then, a few moments later, opened it again and read more closely. Then he looked away again. He had found the grieving heart of the entire problem. Expecting to wade into a tentative, accusatory stream of complaints that would sound boringly familiar, he instead found himself swept up in an ocean of suffering and frustration. It was much like the organization meetings: Here was a son who was refused dental treatment for an abscessed tooth until the pain became so great he committed suicide. Here was a daughter who became addicted to street drugs while in the hospital. Here was a brother with unexplained broken bones. Here was a sister prematurely discharged and lost to the streets.

But this document went beyond the anguish of the meetings. These pages contained in no uncertain detail every problem Alex was aware of, and then some. It was more than a catalog of pain. These relatives knew what could be expected of a good hospital, and so they knew how to criticize a bad one. Everything was there:

The existence of premature discharge and treatment by bus and plane ticket was not a matter of debate for them. They knew it existed because their loved ones had disappeared from the hospital and never been heard from again.

They knew all the filthy corners of the hospital that never seemed to get clean, all the ancient equipment and furniture that was never replaced or repaired.

They measured the adequacy of the food by the frequency of food poisonings as well as by the lack of nutritional counseling.

The name of every psychiatrist who had no time for supportive psychotherapy and who only supervised medications was known to them.

They knew all the areas where staff was undertrained and at least a quarter-century behind the times.

All the wards where constructive and recreational activities consisted of television, cigarettes, and coffee were listed, as well as those where these items were used as punishment-reward incentives.

They knew which doors were supposed to be locked and hardly ever were, and which doors were never to be locked, in case of emergency, but always were.

The fact that the administrative structure of the hospital was a shambles was no secret to them because they could never find anyone who would take responsibility for anything.

They knew that medical protocols were not being followed because their sons and daughters and mothers and fathers were moved from unit to unit with little or no continuity of treatment, not to mention psychiatric justification.

They didn't need a grand jury investigation to know that illegal drugs were being sold or traded for sex and other favors, because their children were the addicts and the victims.

They didn't need to read the journals to find out about the controversy over whether caffeine stimulated behavioral problems in patients: Their relatives were on both sides of the violence.

They had a precise list of the treatable medical diseases that went untreated, the mysterious broken bones, the unexplained deaths.

Every night they forced themselves to sleep with the knowledge that their loved ones were living in old buildings with decrepit or inoperable fire alarms, and that staff and patients had never practiced emergency evacuation.

Parents didn't need psychiatric training to know that medications their children were receiving were often changed without adequate justification or monitoring—they witnessed the seizures, the decompensations, the overdoses.

The Centers for Disease Control didn't have to tell them that precautions against AIDS infections were inadequate, because their loved ones told them about the fights they had with HIV carriers.

They didn't need the unions to tell them that morale was poor among staff members. They knew that discipline was spotty and that often the best workers were laid off while it was next to impossible to get sadistic staff members fired.

They felt only too harshly the frustration of trying to deal with an unyielding bureaucracy run as if it were a clandestine military exercise. If they couldn't have a voice in the proceedings, they at least wanted an ear—just to know what was going on with their children, their parents, their aunts and uncles and cousins. Just to know what they had to do to try to get them seen by a medical doctor or dentist, or find out who they had to talk to in order to get permission to take their relative home for a weekend.

Most of all, they knew the high premium put on silent acquiescence, because their relatives were the ones who were harassed, beaten, provoked, mistreated, and arbitrarily punished when they complained to hospital staff.

This became, for Alex, a crucial detail. The Organization families poured forth the facts in this amazing document only because their anonymity had been guaranteed. They knew too well that retaliations would fall upon those least able to defend themselves—the patients.

This was a problem because Alex had realized he wanted the Family Organization to testify to the accreditation committee when it visited Bedloe again in September. And that's what he had told Fran Channing when he called her after reading the report, waking her and her husband.

But what about his own silence? What was the value of Alex's acquiescence?

For now Alex felt suspended between two versions of himself. One Alex Greco was the man who took on the world and did not bow, the warrior physician, the marine who went up the bore against enemy fire. This Alex Greco was born of a time in Alex's life when everyone he loved in his life was alive and well, when sickness was something he studied in medical school and treated from the safe distance provided by his enthusiasm and belief, a time when the smile on the face of a beautiful woman meant only the possibility of love, a time before he knew all the ways in which the slimy beasts of mortality could crawl into the foundations of a man's life and eat.

Enthusiasm, Alex knew, was derived from words that meant "with the gods." He had not been with the gods for a long time. Now that he had emptied himself before the Family Organization in the basement of the church, he did not even have the fullness of his suffering to harbor as a secret burden of heroism. He was one sufferer among many. There was nothing special about his war. Alex was a citizen of a devastated city, one of many survivors wandering through the bombed-out streets counting the maimed and dead, hoarding their anguish not out of greed or fear, but because there was no clear perpetrator, unless mortality itself could be said to have intent.

This is the way a man splits: His youthful energy is a freight train. It can be sent to different tracks, even derailed, but it takes many years to deplete such an elemental force. Youthful purpose is something else. It is the most delicate of armors and is easily separated from the engine that gives it such glory. It is bartered, sold for time and gambled for advantage, traded for the paraphernalia of success and power. Alex had spent his slowly, making the compromises the world demanded, telling himself that compromise was the currency of a successful life. But compromise was a paper currency backed by the precious metal of Alex's heart, and his creditors had slowly made their claims.

But there was always plenty of paper to be printed. There was always plenty of room in the world's cash registers for compromise.

So here was the other Alex Greco, the successful physician, the medical director of one of the largest mental hospitals in the world, the man whose golden youth had bought a sterling career, but which now had the cold inhuman loneliness of brass. But brass was a valuable commodity, still, and frankly, much more practical in the real world.

There were decisions to be made. Sam Akbar had summoned Alex to his office. The accreditation committee's visit to Bedloe was one month away, and there was work to be done. That's the way the meeting had begun, predictably enough. One version of Alex was ready to deal with Akbar. He knew what was coming, certain compromises here and there. Now Alex would find out why Sam had not made more trouble over the reforms in D-7. At Bedloe, all silence, all acquiescence had a price.

"Uh, yeah, Alex, the damn committee thing coming up," Sam muttered, letting Alex know why he was there.

Alex nodded but kept silent.

Akbar wasn't watching him, however, He had turned his chair slightly and was staring out the window.

"We're gonna make it past those dickheads this time."

Alex inspected Sam, knowing he should be accustomed to the man's vulgarity by this time, but still feeling pinched by it.

"We've got nothing to worry about," Sam declared.

"Did you read the Family Organization report?" Alex asked calmly, referring to the copy Fran and the other members of the Organization had dropped off at their unexpectedly brief meeting with Sam at the end of July.

Sam waved his hand through the air as if dispelling an offensive odor. "That piece of crap! I chucked it."

"You think that was a good idea?"

"Who gives a shit about them? Look, I've dealt with these people before. Some parent gets all pissed off because her kid goes nuts and the whole mess of them get riled up. They start bitching all over the place. Best course of action is to ignore them. They get tired and give up before you know it."

Sam drummed his fingers on his desk, just short of slamming his palm down for emphasis. "Know what I mean?"

Alex nodded. More than anything he wanted to escape, to look out the window and follow the path his eyes made through the lush jungle of bushes, flowers, and trees outside Sam's office.

Sam turned and their eyes met and held on. "We've gotta get together on this committee business, Alex," Akbar declared.

Then Sam proceeded to tell Alex what he assumed they agreed upon. It was a list of all the major issues of care in which Alex had pressed for more reform. Although it began with the few matters in which Alex had enjoyed Sam's grudging cooperation, it soon found its way into the areas where Sam had steadfastly resisted making substantial changes.

"You're gonna be a team player, right?" Sam had finally said. "Otherwise those bastards'll close the goddamn hospital."

Never before in his life had Alex been conscious of trying to keep his head perfectly still so as not to indicate any feeling or acknowledge any response. He was being asked to lie, not outright, but by silence, by collegial complicity, by the earnest forgetfulness of a "team" that certainly wasn't doing anywhere near its best. He was being asked to join a conspiracy of mediocrity.

No, Alex realized, he had joined it long ago. He was being asked to assert that mediocrity was the best he could do.

Alex walked out of Akbar's office not sure of whether he succeeded in erasing the grimace from his face. Fortunately, it was a short walk to his own sanctuary, and no one saw him in the hall.

29 _____

For weeks, Alex tried to reduce his dilemma to a simple question: *I do this, or I do this*. But when a man is suspended between two versions of himself, and he cannot find a compromise, then he is forced to abandon one version. Alex had made his way this far by keeping the one version in sight while adopting the other. He knew that this time he would have to abandon one or the other.

Alex made his decision on one of those days in August that is still strong with summer's heat, but which is caressed by the tender coolness of fall. Wilson Cottage was having a picnic and barbecue at Poe Lake, and Alex had been invited. It would give him the opportunity to tell Doc his decision.

There wasn't much of a parking lot at Poe Lake, just a place on the side of the road where the state had spread some gravel years ago. Grass grew up through the stones here and there. Alex pulled in and parked between Wendy's truck and Doc's old Buick. A couple of cars he didn't recognize and a hospital van were parked under a tree.

The air was lighter and cooler up here. Two miles from the

administration building and maybe a thousand feet of elevation made a difference of five to ten degrees this time of year. Alex took a deep breath. Something had come across his desk a year ago about the state's wanting to sell off several hundred acres near the lake. Fortunately, the economy of the area had seen its best years long ago. Nevertheless, several real estate agents had been contacted, and a few had salivated at the prospect of leveling every tree for two hundred acres and installing condominiums.

Alex smelled the barbecue and heard the sing-song voices. The exaggerated laughter of a patient rose above the others. Most of the party was buzzing on the flat terrace in front of the cabin.

"Why hello, Dr. Alex Greco."

Alex turned on the path. Behind him, a tall, masculine-looking woman with short blond hair was walking up from the lake with a pert younger woman with close-cropped brown hair. Both women seemed to carry themselves slowly and methodically, with solemnity out of place in these surroundings. Alex recognized the tall patient as Paula Frickel—who demanded that she be called Sister Matthew. She was a bonafide nun, whose diagnosis was schizoaffective. Doc thought she had a healthy dose of personality disorders, too, principally of the psychopathic variety. Sister Matthew was known to sexually take advantage of younger female patients. Alex knew that plenty of sex went on among the patients, and that it was generally tolerated by the staff. But Sister Matthew's favors tended toward the sadomasochistic, and the Wilson Cottage staff had their hands full trying to keep her from hurting the patients who couldn't defend themselves.

Sister Matthew wasn't at Bedloe for her sexual practices. She had gone home one Easter and beaten her mother to death with a crucifix. Doc suspected the woman was still running her convent from the hospital. Every now and then a gaggle of nuns visited Wilson Cottage and had a big meeting with her. Doc was stymied by this patient, who was usually in total control of every therapy session, which then went nowhere. As far as she was concerned, she committed a terrible sin, but confessed it—to a bishop, Doc always pointed out—and was forgiven. Beyond that, she wouldn't give an inch, and medications couldn't budge her.

The nun addressed Alex as if he were a subordinate. According to

Doc, this patient addressed everyone that way. Sure enough, she wore the self-sure smile of someone accustomed to getting her way.

The woman accompanying her Alex recognized as Dorothy Weston, a young mother who, in the grip of postpartum psychosis had tried to kill her newborn daughter. The baby survived and was now in grammar school, but after several years at Bedloe Dorothy just wasn't responding to treatment. According to Doc, her husband brought the kids to visit her twice a month.

Dorothy was holding her own, Doc had reported. At this moment, however, she looked to Alex like her grip had loosened. Her eyes, when she allowed Alex to get a look at them, were vacant and red at the same time. She kept two steps behind the larger woman, and appeared frightened by the encounter. She reached up toward Sister Matthew's thick bare arm, but then withdrew the hand.

"Hello, Sister," he nodded. "Are you enjoying yourself?"

"Yes, Doctor, I am. The Lord has blessed us with this wonderful day, hasn't He?"

Alex nodded and smiled and walked on, faster, away from the two women and toward the terrace, away from his thoughts on sin and redemption. Perhaps Sister Matthew's ministrations would help Dorothy Weston expiate what Doc's drugs and therapy could not. Alex doubted it.

There was a time when both women might have been burned as witches, although Alex figured the religious court would probably have been as frustrated with Sister Matthew as modern psychiatry was.

Psychopaths were as fascinating as they were deadly. All the world's great murderers and politicians had a big dose of it. Sam Akbar had a touch of it, a man so angry and mean-spirited could not have achieved such a position of power unless significant portions of his brain were specifically designed to manipulate people and, without a trace of conscience, use them for his own ends—even if it meant their suffering. Sometimes, especially if it meant their suffering.

Some professionals believed psychopaths were "created" by abusive parents. Alex believed that abuse might precipitate a disorder, but he was convinced that no parent, no matter how inept or cruel, could create a true psychopath.

Alex knew we all had a touch of it. How else to explain the suffering we closed our eyes on every day?

The path took him closer to the lake for a stretch. A young man, whom Alex recognized as Tom Coolidge, one of Wilson Cottage's bipolar, or manic-depressive, patients, was sitting on a rock throwing pebbles into the water. Tom waved, and Alex smiled and waved back. Up ahead, he saw Doc standing in the middle of the crowd. Some of the people next to Doc saw Alex and pointed at him. Alex waved.

"Well," Doc said, "our esteemed medical director has graced us with his presence. Hello, Dr. Greco!"

Henry Dove, wearing a tall white chef's cap, was stabbing and shuffling hot dogs on the grill. Next to him, on the food table, there was a tall pile of cooked hot dogs. As he added to the pile, Wendy, wearing a wider, looser chef's hat that kept flopping in front of her face, inserted hot dogs into buns and placed them on a plate. "I think that's enough for now, Henry, dear. Just about everybody's eaten."

"Well, there are two more packages here. They'll spoil if we don't cook them," Henry said and attacked the grill with renewed vigor.

Wendy brushed the big white hat back and, when her eyes met Alex's, rolled them skyward for an instant. "Hi, Doctor Greco. I'm glad you could make it. Have a hot dog. Henry has done a marvelous job."

Doc nodded. "They are perfect specimens. Just right. This man has done this before, Alex."

Alex noticed a bittersweet smile flash across Henry Dove's face. Henry had a wife and children at one time, friends, family, business associates. There would have been barbecues in that prior life.

"I made the potato salad, Dr. Greco. Try it," Wendy said. The frail Lily Speere was standing next to her.

"I . . . I h-helped," Lily said, more to Wendy than to Alex.

"Lily peeled the potatoes and sliced the celery. That's right," Wendy smiled broadly.

"Try the relish on that," Wendy said to Alex as he accepted the hot dog she served him in a bun. "Lily sliced the pickles herself."

Lily blushed and bowed her head even lower.

"Try some of this fruit salad," Ramona Lopez chimed. "Me and Patty Robito made it." The chubby patient smiled at Alex and her eyes twinkled. Ramona had once been a nurse at Valley Hospital, but had lost her job when it was discovered that she had wheeled several patients into the operating room—for the wrong operations. That was during the manic phase of her disease. During the depressed phase, after losing her job, she tried to kill herself.

"It's great," Doc confirmed. "They were slicing fruit all night. Well worth the effort."

On the other side of the terrace, a group of patients sitting on stone benches started singing "Row Row Row Your Boat," in rounds, led by Bennett Ackerman, proudly sporting his red cowboy hat. Alex had been just about to ask where Patty Robito was, when he noticed the attractive young woman with long, straight brown hair among the singing group. Patty's diagnosis was bipolar, but Doc said she was mainly depressed. She seemed to respond well to treatment, except she always lost ground every other week when her husband arrived for a conjugal visit. He picked her up after supper, took her to a cheap motel for a couple of hours, and then dropped her back at the hospital. Wendy said Patty would stand there waving goodbye for half an hour after he left. Then she'd be sick for a week and everyone in the unit would have to keep an eye on her.

Alex returned Patty's wave and smiled.

"Where's our distinguished resident physician?" Alex asked Doc.

Wendy smiled, then wrestled the smile into a grimace. Doc saw her and cleared his throat. "Well, last we saw him he was having a heart-to-heart discussion with Ethel Flynn, our distinguished pregnant patient."

"I think they went off into the woods, Doc," Wendy hastened to add, as if Doc knew but didn't want to say it out loud.

"Yes. Well . . . the woods are beautiful."

Alex raised his eyebrows for Wendy's benefit, giving her the acknowledgment she was waiting for. But he already knew of Doc's concern for Rosey. Doc had taken Rosey aside and given him, "the standard three-dollar lecture on getting too close to patients and how it messes everything up." But Rosey had simply turned it back on Doc and accused him of acting like a father with Lily Speere and others.

"That's the idea," Doc had said. "But a father is different from a big brother. Or a friend. Or a lover." Doc complained to Alex that he sometimes felt that he hadn't only lost a resident psychiatrist, but had gained an additional patient.

"I made the cupcakes, Dr. Greco," Wendy said. Alex knew this was an invitation, so he picked one up and smiled at Wendy.

"You don't want to miss one of Wendy's cupcakes," the blond man who was now standing next to her said. Alex knew the man's face, but couldn't recognize him as one of Wilson Cottage's patients or staff.

"Dr. Greco," Wendy interrupted his confusion, "this is Dan Billings."

"Of course, Dan. You're the new psychologist in D-7." Alex noticed that Dan's eyes didn't seem to be able to stray very long from Wendy. For her part, Wendy stole glances at Dan only when she thought no one, particularly Dan, was watching.

When Alex had dutifully eaten at least one of everything prepared by the staff and patients of Wilson Cottage, he took a deep breath and caught Doc's eyes with his own. "I need a walk," he nodded.

On their way down the path, Alex noticed that the lake shimmered with purple ripples in the early evening light.

"Getting dark sooner now," Doc grunted.

Alex took a deep breath. "Making up my mind hasn't lightened me," he said.

"You expected a burden to be removed?"

"I don't know."

"Making the decision is just loading the gun, Alex. You've decided what kind of ammunition, that's all. Scattershot or bullets. You've still got to take your shot. Did you tell Sam?"

Alex nodded.

"How do you tell a man what you told him? That's something I don't think I know how to do."

"I just told him we have some significant differences, and I believed I couldn't ignore these differences when the committee was here. That's all."

"You told him you're not playing on his team, right?" Doc smiled, and the quality of Doc's smile annoyed Alex. He seemed to relish the showdown.

"What'd he say, Alex?"

"He asked for my resignation."

[2]

On their way back up the path, Doc and Alex came upon a schizophrenic patient who was about to be discharged back to the county. Robert Bullman, a short man with long, thinning gray hair, was sitting in the middle of a group of three patients and one psych tech. Alex knew his prognosis was not good, since Robert didn't like to take his medications. But his county was getting stingy and Robert was headed for the bus station.

Robert knew it, too. "I'm gonna jump on a bus and go to California. I been waiting for my chance. No way I'm goin' back home, no way. I think my father and mother live in California. Or Ohio. I'm goin'. They kick me outta this place, I'm takin' off, that's all. Say goodbye to Robert Bullman."

They walked away, back toward the terrace, where a line of colored lanterns strung over the heads of Wendy, Dan, Lily and the others had come on. The entire group was singing, led by the man with no head.

30

In the weeks before the National Medical Accreditation Committee arrived at Bedloe, swarms of carpenters, electricians, painters, plumbers, and janitors came out of hiding and fulfilled repair requests and work orders that had been lying unacknowledged for months, even years.

Wilson Cottage received its share of belated attention from the hospital maintenance department, beginning with a new coat of paint. A hole in the wall with wires sticking out behind a sofa was diagnosed by electricians as the remnants of an electrical outlet that had long been torn out. Scorch marks on the wires indicated that someone had shorted them, perhaps in an attempt to start a fire. In any case, the fuse had blown—which explained why the ceiling light in Doc's office never worked. The wires were capped, the hole plastered over, and the fuse replaced.

D-7, one of the neediest units, got new light fixtures, new paint on the walls, new locks on broken doors, new leather restraint straps for the seclusion rooms, new tiles in the bathroom to replace those which had been picked loose and ferreted away by patients, a new toilet, new doors on the toilet stalls to replace those which had been torn off so long ago that no one knew when or why it had happened, a rebuilt air conditioner, and new windows to replace the cardboard put up by psych techs after the glass had been broken. The renaissance of D-7 continued despite the intrusions of carpenters and other workers. But as much as the staff was doing, they knew they weren't doing enough.

[2]

On the day the accreditation committee arrived at Bedloe, the only traces of the recent invasion of workmen were the splashes of paint here and there in the grass, and these were removed as soon as the carpenters, electricians, plumbers, janitors, and painters could exchange their tools for lawn mowers. The hospital gleamed.

But the men and women of the committee had seen gleaming hospitals before. They may have nodded and shaken hands with Sam Akbar and Alex Greco and others as they entered the hospital. They may even have smiled. But their eyes were saving their real hunger for the records. In the reams of hospital paperwork they would find the true signature of Bedloe State Hospital. The committee would open the books and ask this question over and over again: *Is Procedure being followed?* This question was the commander in chief, and its power radiated down through dozens of more specific questions about the way things were done at the hospital:

Were doctors hired properly? Were their credentials checked out adequately? Was their performance monitored?

Was the medical staff organized?

Was the administration of the hospital responsive to the medical staff?

Were medication records adequate? Were drugs being given for appropriate reasons? Were risks and benefits adequately considered?

Were procedures instituted, followed, and monitored in lab workups, exams, emergency care, and other medical areas?

Were hospital-caused infections recorded and controlled?

Were the hospital buildings and grounds safe?

Were medical records clear, complete, and accurate?

Were standard psychiatric procedures being followed with regard to restraint and seclusion?

Were patients adequately assessed for danger to self or others? Were suicidal patients adequately managed?

Were violent incidents properly handled, investigated, and recorded? Was assaultive behavior properly managed?

Were patients missing?

Were patients involved in illegal activities either on or off grounds?

Were patients in possession of nonprescribed controlled substances, alcohol, or weapons?

Were treatment plans individualized and carried out for each patient? Were treatment goals being met?

Was medical-surgical care of psychiatric patients adequate? Were patients developing physical problems in the hospital, such as bedsores, infections, pneumonia, and traumatic injuries?

Were patients admitted and discharged for the proper reasons? Was there any evidence of patients kept too long or discharged too soon?

Were the lines of communication, responsibility, and authority clear?

Were deaths adequately investigated?

Over the several days of studying Bedloe's records for answers to these and other questions, the accreditation committee members gradually lost their polite, collegial smiles. By the end of the third day, they were giving only perfunctory nods to physicians or administrators. They had to send a staff assistant out for more notepads four times in the nine days they reviewed Bedloe's records.

The actual inspections of the hospital were postponed first for a day, then for a week. Three washers and two dryers broke down in the hospital laundry because, expecting the committee to visit, the wards were sending linens and clothes back in two-day cycles instead of the usual four. The groundskeepers raked in a week's worth of overtime mowing the lawns every third day, and one of the hospital's water pumps broke, they were watering so much. Timothy Buck stayed until midnight helping the mechanic fix the pump, since this was the one that supplied the farm with water for irrigation.

Finally, the inspection team took off their glasses, rubbed their eyes, and walked out of the conference rooms where they had been examining records for almost two weeks. The hospital stood at attention before them.

Several patients saw the inspection team's visit as an opportunity to redress grievances. Some were convinced the team was sent there for some special purpose specifically having to do with their release or recognition as not ill and imprisoned at Bedloe under false pretenses. One man in D-7 confronted the team with the information that he was, in fact, the Savior and he was damn glad somebody had come looking for him. Two patients in the V-unit tried to make a deal with George Konopski to be on their best behavior in exchange for an extra pack of cigarettes.

After four days walking around the hospital, the inspection team was done. They retired to their conference room to prepare their questions for what was politely termed the "exit interview," but which was actually a wholesale barbecue in which the chef cross-examined the live meat while the heat was searing its juices.

Flames of varying intensity were applied to various members of the hospital staff. Some witnesses were not roasted at all, but were actually served cake. The hottest flames were reserved for the administration, which had to answer for whatever litany of faults the team had composed for the occasion.

In Bedloe's case, an opera—no, an entire liturgical calendar of operas—could have been written around the problems uncovered by the committee.

Although much improvement had been made in morale and performance of duties by the medical staff, not all psychiatrists were found to be performing at a professional level. The Dean Lester case was given extra scrutiny by the committee. This was the first place that Alex's testimony and Sam Akbar's diverged. In a closed, individual session, Akbar told the committee that he had pointed out conditions in Lester's unit more than a year before, but he had done so informally, not wishing to "stir up trouble among the psychiatrists." In a similar private interview, Alex told the committee that he had encountered resistance from Akbar in cleaning up D-7, and he had the unanswered memos to prove it.

Lester was not the only psychiatrist found wanting, however. Alex was praised for his work in organizing the medical staff and invigo-rating its morale. Nevertheless, there were still a few physicians not operating in a manner consistent with their training and the privi-leges granted. In a few units there were no planned programs of psychiatric therapy. Medical treatment often seemed to be on a "by crisis only" basis. There were no records of routine exams and many of the admissions to the infirmary were for conditions that might have been prevented. In a few instances, the unit physician appeared to have only vaguely paid attention to matters of quality care.

Not all such infractions were attributable to psychiatrists, since most units were directed by other professionals and it was up to the unit supervisor to make sure that some form of therapy was planned and carried out. In wards where staff felt overburdened, there was a tendency to let such plans slip away as day-to-day matters demanded attention. The committee was not necessarily looking for a perfectly organized and executed daily program of therapy. They knew that in many cases just keeping the patients clean, fed, and occupied in some peaceful manner demanded con-stant effort. Nevertheless, they wanted to see evidence that the staff at least acknowledged that the hospital was not a human warehouse.

[3]

Despite the armada of words launched by the accreditation com-mittee, the quality of care in a mental hospital is not a matter of rules and bylaws, but a matter of organization of human emotions. Human will can be applied, like a stick to a herd of beasts, but attitude is what steers. And how do you describe attitude: *Staff shall at all times cheerfully demonstrate a deeply caring and humane attitude toward all patients?*

The committee, unofficially—for there were no words written directly for this purpose—was aware that Bedloe State Hospital's attitude was suffering.

The role of the leader is not only to make sure that attention is paid to details, but to determine the attitude, to call out the attitude every day so that no one will forget it. This is how attitude is kept healthy and vigorous in an institution. It is called morale, esprit de corps, team spirit. It is how the individual mind, alone with itself, views and accepts and executes its responsibilities to the group. The psych tech who may never have a conversation with the superintendent of the hospital will respond to the attitude of the leader nevertheless. He may not even know what that leader's attitude is, but he will live it every working moment, because it will be in the wind and waves all around him.

At Bedloe there was a conflict of attitudes, and the committee could see it in the paperwork, in the data, in the epic battles fought by battalions of words. They could see Alex's slow progress at instilling a sense of professional pride among the psychiatrists, see it in the increasing frequency of medical decisions signed with a sure hand in dark, indelible ink. And then there was Sam Akbar's signature, more often denying something than approving.

[4]

As a prelude to the session in which both Sam and Alex would appear, others were given their chance before the committee. Doc Rush was not a man to climb aboard a soapbox, but he spoke his mind when asked. That Doc was impatient with the entire parade of inspectors became clear very early.

"I was trained in an era when you were considered to have done your job if the patient left the office feeling better than when he came in," Doc began. "It feels like we're treating the charts, not the patients. If I want to change a drug a patient is getting, for example, I not only have to mark the chart, which is fine, but I have to fill out three different forms so three different bureaucracies can look over my shoulder. Believe me, it often comes down to a decision of whether to do what I think is best for the patient or whether it is really worth the extra trouble."

The committee knew beforehand that Doc had apparently settled that dilemma. The records of his patients that came from other more bureaucratically responsible members of the treatment team showed that Doc's patients were among the best cared for in the hospital. Doc's own paperwork was always a study in minimalism, and it was always late.

Doc's comments on the committee's investigation were only an introduction to what he was really there to do, which was to deliver a stunning, though gentlemanly criticism of the way Sam Akbar was running the hospital. "Morale just isn't what it ought to be around this hospital," Doc said, "and there's no excuse for it. It doesn't matter how much money you have to work with or how sick your patients are, you can still have good morale. You can still have people going about their work with enthusiasm, good humor, and some hope that they're helping a little. But that's not the case here, and the responsibility has to go all the way to the top. That's where morale starts, good or bad. And there's a dark cloud over this institution. We're not doing as good a job as we can, as we know how."

[5]

The Family Organization agonized over whether to send representatives to testify before the committee. In the weeks before the special meeting called to make the decision, there were arguments at home as families split over what to do. Members spent long, anguished hours on the telephone with one another describing their fears and their determination to help their relatives. There were hastily arranged sessions with attorneys. Some families revived efforts to have their loved ones transferred from Bedloe to other facilities. Many just sat down together at the kitchen table and went through old photo albums.

Fran Channing was afraid for her son's life. This was not a new experience for her. In the early years, every time he became unmanageable and dashed out the door, Fran knew she might never see Walter alive again, or at all, for that matter. So once she was sure he wasn't just sitting on the lawn taking off his clothes instead of losing himself on the streets, she called the police.

And even that she did with full knowledge that if the wrong police officers found Walter, he could be shot. Over the years, thanks to education programs sponsored by the Family Organization and the police department, the local officers had become better at subduing the mentally ill without violence. But there were frequent incidents where things just became too tense too fast. In the past year two members' sons had been killed by police officers, one locally and one somewhere in the Midwest.

Even if the officers who found him were experienced and took him in with hardly an unkind word, Walter was far from safe in jail. The suicide rate for mentally ill people during the first twenty-four hours of incarceration was too high to bet against. So when Walter was lost, after notifying the police, Fran spent the first few hours driving and scanning the streets where she knew he liked to hang out. But once she was certain she wasn't going to find him, she rushed home and spent the rest of the night on the phone checking with the police so she could either get him home or get him transferred to a county facility right away.

Of course, Walter wasn't exactly safe there, either.

But where was he safe? Nowhere, and over the years all the individual fears had run together into one. Walter's life was not protected by the same customs, laws, or kindnesses most people enjoyed. By virtue of his illness he was exiled to another dimension of our world, a cruel place where the strong pressed every advantage against the weak.

And now, after almost eight months for Walter at Bedloe State Hospital and six months for Fran as a member of the Family Organization, she wondered whether Bedloe wasn't the most dangerous place of all.

Fran had heard the stories of other Organization members, knew how many of them no longer trusted anyone, knew how many had lost faith. The most common themes were that in the weeks after the Organization complained or just communicated with the hospital administration, something happened to their relatives. To be sure, not every child or parent or cousin was affected, and these incidents certainly also happened to patients not connected to the Organization. But they happened often enough and with chilling enough consistency for members to predict:

Normally nonviolent patients would be provoked into an assault or a violent decompensation. At the very least there would be a loss of privileges—no freedom of the hospital grounds, no recreational activities, no dessert, no TV. From there, the punishment escalated all the way from sudden transfer to a more restrictive unit to becoming the victim of one of Bedloe's mysterious never-explained assaults.

One member had been known as a vocal supporter of her son's rights. She had monitored his care diligently and called the hospital often when there were problems. Hers was one of the Organization's success stories. The boy was scheduled to be discharged to a model board-and-care home. But a week before his discharge the normally calm patient was backed into a corner by a psych tech and provoked into a fight. As a result the son was sent to Willowdale, a hospital for violent penal code patients.

All Organization members lived with this knowledge, but they fought on, careful to try as much as possible to frame their complaints in a spirit of cooperation rather than accusation.

That's why the *Report* was such a big step for them, to come forward and articulate the details of the calamities and crimes they and their loved ones lived with every day. Even behind the cloak of anonymity, it was a daring move. The administration knew the names of the Organization members and their relatives who were patients.

And now this Dr. Greco was asking the Organization members to step forward, give their names, and testify before the accreditation committee! He might as well have asked them to sew targets on their loved ones' backs.

Alex had told them he believed that testifying would be a logical extension of the other work the Organization was doing to improve care for the mentally ill. And given the solid stone wall around the administration at the hospital, this was the most vulnerable point at which they could marshal their forces. This was going over the head of not only Sam Akbar but also the state department of mental health.

Fran knew that many members of the Organization didn't know what to make of Alex Greco. The first time they heard him speak, no one could believe what they were hearing. They believed that anyone who spoke out against the system from within would eventually be banished from it. Yet here was a powerful man from the other side of the stone wall who nevertheless seemed to be on their side.

No, it was more than that. Alex Greco did not seem to have abandoned one set of allegiances for another. Their side *was* his side. He wanted the same things they did, and he had not learned these standards from them, but from his own training, experience, and conscience. Good care was good care, whether it was described in an Organization memo or a medical text. Alex's dream was their dream, just as his sorrow and frustration were theirs, too.

But had the psychiatrist gone mad? Didn't he know that he was sewing a target on his own back as well as on theirs?

"Well," Fran had said to some of the other members, "it doesn't matter if we have targets on our backs, because our backs are against the wall."

The actual meeting was uncharacteristically muted at first, perhaps because everyone already knew what the decision would be. Finally the vote was taken, the decision made, and then a nervous silence lay over the room. The energy bound up in each family's apprehension and determination wasn't released until they took up the next and last order of business. A merry boisterousness took over as they arranged car pools to the hospital for the day they would all testify.

So dozens of these families, most of whom had first approached Bedloe State Hospital alone, fearful, intimidated, drove up to its administration building in a caravan of crowded cars. There would always be sorrows and terrors each mother and father and child and sibling would have to bear alone, but on that day no one was alone. They were an army of defiance and were not to be denied.

The first speaker from the group, Fran Channing, hastened to go on record by prefacing their testimony with the statement that all members feared for the safety of their relatives, not only from the day-to-day situations that developed because of the way the hospital was run, but also from reprisals related to their speaking out to the committee. "Though we are afraid for our children and other family members," Fran said, "we feel it is important enough to take this chance and speak out to you." She then proceeded to begin reading her portion of the Organization's detailed report of complaints against Bedloe State Hospital. Because her son had been a patient for only eight months, Fran's list was relatively short. Members who came later spoke much longer.

The voices broken with emotion cast an attentive silence over the room. Though they did not address the conflict between Sam and Alex, the parents were generally critical of the way the hospital was run, though a few of them praised Alex Greco and the improvements he had brought. They reserved their most careful language for accounts of the meeting with Sam in which he had rejected their pleas for reform. And when the last member had testified, the room was silent for a long time.

[6]

When Akbar had asked for his resignation, Alex was thrown into confusion—but only for a few hours. A walk with Maria across the ballpark and a good night's sleep calmed him. The next morning he went in to the hospital early, in case Akbar had plans to lock him out of his office, and called the state department of mental health. Alex spoke to the director of mental health for the state and told him, simply, that the superintendent of the hospital had asked for his resignation.

"What the hell for?" Bill Crockett asked. Bill, a psychiatrist who was good enough as a physician but who found his true calling in politics, was in the middle of a congressional battle to merge the department of mental health with the state's services for drug addiction. Though advocates for the mentally ill saw this as pure politics that would further deteriorate care, Crockett's supporters figured the mentally ill would benefit from the society's current phobia for drug addiction. Though Bill now had to justify every penny spent for the mentally ill, no one minded voting more money for the battle against drugs. Alex thought of it as a meaningless political squabble, since roughly half of the mentally ill were addicted anyway.

After Alex told Bill about his meeting with Sam, there was a moment of silence, a perfect silence, Alex thought, in which Bill did not breath faster, did not sigh, did not give the slightest indication of how the information had affected him. Just a blank space, which Alex was about to fill by asking, "What do you want me to do?"

But Alex didn't have to ask that question. Bill said, "This is a hell of a time for this."

Alex, when going over the conversation, realized that these first words out of Bill Crockett's mouth were not an expression of exasperation, but were the width and breadth of his logic, a statement of his justification. Then Bill said, "Ignore the request, Alex. I'll speak to Sam."

Later that afternoon, Bill called Alex and told him that, as far as the state department of mental health was concerned, a request for Alex's resignation had never been made and that Alex should consider it that way, too.

Alex felt even more threatened than before, and accused himself of paranoia all the way home that afternoon. Akbar had disappeared from the hospital at lunchtime. Alex realized that this was a bigger game than any conflict between him and Akbar. What bothered Alex was the conviction that Crockett was not explaining everything to him, and that after his brief call the state official must have spent considerably more time on the phone with Akbar.

This is a hell of a time for this, Alex thought, and mulled Crockett's statement over and over. For the time being, Alex realized, the state had no choice but to keep him as medical director. He was sure that Crockett must have grilled Akbar over whether there was really an issue strong enough to fire Alex just days before the committee would show up. Administrative disarray was a major black mark against a hospital. Crockett knew that the committee would be sure to call Alex in for testimony, regardless of how strong a case Akbar had for his dismissal. Nothing could be gained by dismissing Alex, and much could be lost. So Crockett moved to delete the request.

But if this was not the time, when was?

[7]

The committee did not put Alex and Sam face to face until near the end of the hearing. Since Sam and Alex were the two people most responsible for the hospital, they received the full verbal grilling.

When the committee brought Sam and Alex together at last, they could see the conflict in the way the two men were uncomfortable in the same room together: Both seemed to be making a great effort to appear confident and relaxed, but only Akbar was, also with effort, smiling. Alex's face was securely set in the somber calm of the warrior, beyond confidence, beyond fear, accepting that he was fighting for something beyond his life, but for his life, too.

Alex told the committee that there were many fundamental disagreements between him and the superintendent on matters directly and tangentially related to patient care. His most damning criticism was that the lines of authority in the hospital were still vaguely defined and that patient care ultimately suffered because of the confusion and lack of any effective due process for administrative review. Alex did not directly criticize Sam. Instead, he stated that the hospital would benefit if policy decisions were made with a sympathetic eye toward medical considerations. He listed several reforms that would result in almost immediate improvement in patient care. "You cannot restore health in a toxic atmosphere," he concluded.

Sam seemed to ignore Alex's testimony. During most of it he was involved in a whispered conversation with his secretary. When his turn came, he smiled nervously, and launched into a long list of the improvements he had made at Bedloe State Hospital. When the committee read him a list of the specific problems they had encountered in the records and through their investigation, Sam blamed "other departments."

When the committee pressed for an explanation, Sam blamed the office of the medical director. "As a matter of fact," he said seriously, "I have already asked for the medical director's resignation."

Although other members of the committee calmly made notes, the interrogator did not blink at the revelation, but rather asked Sam whether he believed that someone who was not a physician or who had never been involved in patient care could fully administrate a hospital.

Sam blinked and smiled and answered, "Most of what you need to know is administrative and has nothing to do with clinical issues."

The committee insisted that there was nothing in a hospital that did not touch on clinical issues in some way.

"Well," Sam explained casually, "you can get all the clinical stuff from the book."

The room buzzed and the committee could be seen to raise its collective eyebrows. But in following longstanding tradition and making the interrogation more like a collegial inquiry than a hostile cross-examination, the next few questions were standard ones about administrative procedures.

But then Sam was asked to explain why the rape-murder of Deborah Smith had not been adequately investigated.

Sam hesitated, and in the moments before finally answering, the process of preparing to tell a lie was clearly evident on his face. The committee members put their pencils down.

The next day the committee issued an interim report. The hospital's general probation would continue. Units that had shown sufficient improvement would be provisionally accredited, but full hospital accreditation could not be made until the administration demonstrated a sincere desire to implement the reforms necessary to raise the quality of care. The committee sharply criticized the administration for its style and for thwarting the good intentions of the medical director and other members of the staff. "A mental hospital cannot be run like a covert military operation," the report said. "Morale has suffered and patient care has failed to improve other than through the direct effects of the reforms wrought by the medical director and other staff."

The committee also had sharp words for the state Department of Mental Health for appointing Akbar to this hospital in the first place. "The present superintendent has come from a hospital accredited under less medically stringent standards and was not accustomed to administering a hospital with more demanding medical requirements."

To foster greater cooperation between the superintendent and the medical staff, the committee recommended that the superintendent be a physician.

A reporter covering the accreditation investigation for a local newspaper wrote that it was becoming painfully obvious that the task of running the giant mental hospital was beyond Sam Akbar's capabilities, and that faced with the overwhelming challenge of the hospital, Sam had responded by becoming more restrictive. The result, according to the newspaper article, was "a dark age of management for the hospital, known for coercion, bullying, and insensitivity to the needs of patients and relatives of patients."

Alex had won. He suspected it would not be long before Sam Akbar was gone from the hospital.

31

[1]

In the weeks after the visit of the accreditation committee, Bedloe State Hospital relaxed. Corners that had been kept spotless and shiny regained their dust and grime. Lightbulbs wore out and were not replaced. The groundscrew decided the grass ought to be left alone for a while, since it had been overcut and was turning brown in spots. When windows were broken, cardboard boxes were once again scavenged for pieces to replace the glass.

Word moved through the hospital that Sam Akbar was on his way out. This resulted in a kind of local tension in the vicinity of his office. That Akbar's door should be closed was not unusual. But now there was a dark, vacant quality to the frosted glass. It had not been unusual for Akbar's secretary to tell callers that Akbar was in a meeting and would have to get back to them. But now there was a frenetic, bitter hastiness in the message.

Then one day Akbar was gone from the hospital, promoted to a position in the state department of mental health. After a week of rumors that Alex Greco would be named acting superintendent, a bureaucrat from the state office was installed until a permanent replacement could be found. Alex's boosters among the staff understood the decision not to make him acting superintendent. He was, after all, a party to the conflict. Things had to settle down before he could seriously be considered. Alex was aware of the gossip and tried to ignore it. But on his evening walks with Maria he often brought the conversation around to whether he really wanted the job. Although many physicians take to administrative work with few regrets about leaving clinical work behind, Alex missed working directly with patients. Though he understood he might be able to ultimately accomplish more for the mentally ill as superintendent, he wondered if he could stand being one level further removed from the daily challenges and satisfactions of one-on-one psychiatry.

Alex began another painting, this one of a park, with a baseball diamond in the distance and a grove of trees on top of a hill off to one side. It wasn't until Alex started painting the people in the park in red, white, and blue that he realized he was painting his dream. Somewhat embarrassed at himself and amazed that he felt no discomfort, he continued as faithfully as he could.

[2]

Akbar's departure did not call forth a unanimous sigh of relief. The man had his supporters, who now appeared sullen around the displays of celebration. Nor did his departure result in an immediate revolution at the hospital.

George Konopski enjoyed a respite from the pressure to examine Linus Dillinger. Taking advantage of the lull, he spent more time with his other patients. One morning a new patient showed up at the V-unit and during his entrance interview immediately got down on his knees, pulled on Konopski's coat, and begged for a prescription of tranquilizers. George knew this was a gambit—but the question was which gambit was it, and whose? Patients often begged for drugs, but there was something that didn't smell right about this one. This little man before him was too healthy, too clean. There was not enough dark around his eyes, not enough wrinkles and dirt on his hands. His hair was shaggy but it was a staged kind of shaggy.

His eyes were too clear, and though Konopski saw the predator in them, this predator lacked the nervous line of real fear.

Konopski came to the conclusion that this man was a cop. Maybe he wasn't a fed or a state cop or even a real cop at all. But he was there to trap the doctor.

Regardless of who or what the man was, Konopski was not disposed to write drug prescriptions so easily.

The man continued to beg. Konopski continued to refuse. When the man realized the psychiatrist was not going to give him any drugs, he stood up menacingly and said. "You're not going to write it for me, are you, you son of a bitch?"

Konopski felt the man take a step toward him and, without hesitating or taking his eyes off the patient, rang the bell for the psych techs.

The incident frightened Konopski. He realized that although he had not testified at the committee investigation—on the advice of his attorney—there were people in the administration who wanted to hurt him and that this could have been a set up. He had never been on the receiving end of cold, calculating evil before. He'd worked with murderers and rapists, but always as a professional, the doctor, the one who had power in the situation. He'd had patients attack him, but this was different. Now he believed he was being hunted and, realizing how much damage these people could do, he felt nausea.

[3]

In early October, Dolores Woods went on another shopping expedition to the hospital Central Services Department and brought art supplies back to D-7. She started out big, clearing out the chairs in one of the dayrooms and tacking a giant piece of paper to the wall. Then she gave each of ten patients a box of crayons and sent him to work on his own area of the mural. The patients took to the drawing with enthusiasm, and a few with real talent. Some patients tended to get up close to the paper and scrawl tiny drawings and letters within severely circumscribed spaces. Dolores encouraged them to expand and flex their arms as they made broad and colorful strokes.

Dolores and her charges moved forward musically, too. She liked to use music as a means for expression, to help bring the patients out of the shells, imposed on them by their illnesses. These shells, she learned, were hardened by their brains' difficulties in playing in syncopation with the melodies and rhythms of life. Many, however, had no trouble at all getting in step and in tune with music.

Dolores, with the help of Faith Dundee, began with drum sessions and then graduated to xylophones, bells, and tambourines. She took up to ten patients at a time in these jams, and always had to schedule extra sessions. One patient, with a background in music before he became ill, was able to play entire pieces by Beethoven and Chopin on a small piano that Dolores had wheeled into the unit. Even on his bad days he could play simple nursery songs and a show tune or two. Walter Channing often accompanied Dolores to the Central Services storeroom, and on one occasion the therapist noticed him reverently touching a guitar that was sitting on a shelf.

Even those patients too sick to play an instrument enjoyed dancing. In fact, dancing was becoming so popular around the unit that more than a few patients were beginning to vigorously remind the staff of their promise to invite D-5 over for a party. Finally, Dr. Uyemura, Timothy Buck, and Dan Billings agreed with Faith and Dolores that D-7 was ready for its first "mixer."

They chose Halloween for the event, and set the art classes to work drawing pumpkins and cats. The staff debated for the better part of an hour whether to allow drawings of witches and ghosts. They decided against it, for this year anyway, since it might remind some of the patients of their delusions or spark scary hallucinations. Faith recruited an ad hoc crafts class to make less provocative decorations from corn stalks. The staff and patients of D-5 promised to carve a few pumpkins, while Dolores and a representative of D-5 selected music, to which both units diligently practiced dancing.

To cut down on logistics and food mess, the party was scheduled after supper, with cookies and apple juice to be sent over from the kitchen. In the weeks before Halloween, Faith and Dolores held special social-skills sessions and dance classes, both of which included the etiquette of asking a lady to dance.

On the day of the party, D-7 buzzed like a beehive again—only now the patients who paced were obsessively concerned with the quality of their two-steps. Hands were rubbed together and thrust in and out of pockets in a frenzy of worry over facing down fears many of these men had barely begun to experience when they had become ill. Faith and Dolores and the other staff were fountains of encouragement.

And when the evening finally got underway, Tim remarked to Dolores that, from a certain distance, the whole affair did not appear very different from a junior-high-school dance. There were some real swingers who danced every dance with a different partner. There were some wallflowers of both sexes. There were stiff, self-conscious dancers as well as dancers of the clumsy-but-who-cares variety. There were young ladies who danced with other young ladies, and there were the bashful boys who overcame their fears and asked their favorite girls to dance. There were the coquettish young ladies who blushed and extended their hands—and then danced as if it were the only thing in the world worth doing. Some party-goers stood by the refreshments sipping apple juice and commenting on the skills of the dancers. Others lost themselves in the cookies and hardly ever looked a person of the opposite sex in the eye. Not too much apple juice was spilled, but some was. Not too many cookies or hearts were broken, but some were. Romance blossomed and wilted and blossomed again hundreds of times during the hour and a half.

When it was all over, the staff of D-7 and the staff of D-5 agreed they had started something they did not know how to stop, for several patients were already demanding that the two units do it again. Walter Channing said "I'm ready for this anytime. Once a week, how about it?"

October was the scene of another D-7 victory. The staff had been so impressed with the way the patients handled themselves on the basketball court, the softball field, and around the volleyball net that they decided at the last minute to field a team in the hospital's version of the olympic games. However devastating their illnesses had been to their ability to coordinate both sensory and social input as well as motor output, it was always amazing to see how much of that coordination could be restored by a major dose of competition. Patients who had trouble lifting a forkful of peas to their mouth were seen throwing baskets. Patients who the day before put shoes on the wrong feet were seen swinging the softball bat from both sides of the plate and connecting for extra-base hits. Patients who occasionally had to be restrained from smacking their neighbor at the dinner table were the stars of smacking the volleyball over the net.

D-7 left the field with slightly more than its share of medals, amidst talk by staff of other units of "breaking up the dynasty."

October was a good month for D-7, a month when Faith started sneaking out at night when her shift was over, because she couldn't stand to say good night and leave behind the patients who would still crowd around her and follow her toward the door and want more of what she had given them. And for the same reason, it was a month when Dolores started making a point of saying goodnight quite definitively, believing that the ability to say goodbye was a social skill. It was another month when the entire staff of D-7 realized that as much as they had done, they hadn't done enough.

[4]

Although Alex was not made acting superintendent, he was given more authority. The committee had recommended that the medical director be given line authority in the hospital, which meant that he would have some responsibility in areas other than medical. With this new power, Alex began to bring about some other changes at the hospital. He moved to bring the administration of medical matters more into line with the accreditation committee's standards, and opened the doors of the hospital to patients' family members. He initiated regular meetings between the Family Organization and the administration to discuss the concerns of the relatives and arranged to have a member of the Organization sit on the committee which reviewed all hospital policies and procedures.

Alex knew that even before Sam Akbar left and Bedloe State Hospital began to open up, Timothy Buck and Faith Dundee had plotted to subvert the restrictions that kept the patients' relatives beyond the hospital walls. With Akbar gone, there was no need for secrecy, so D-7 went public: They invited family into the unit. Visiting hours had already been expanded, but D-7 went beyond that. Relative of patients were provided with explanations of how the unit operated, the chain of responsibility, and the phone numbers they might need to get information or services. Tim obtained consent forms from all the patients and sent letters to all family members asking if they wanted to be involved in treatment and other decisions. Some relatives did not, but most did.

Finally, a D-7 open house was planned for the day after Thanksgiving, and all relatives were invited.

Alex extended a similar program throughout the hospital: Parents and other relatives were allowed to attend treatment-team conferences where they were not only informed, but were also consulted on therapy and progress. Relatives were also invited to participate in parties, picnics, barbecues, and other "open house" activities.

At a meeting with the Family Organization, Fran Channing told Alex that the organization was going to mount a letter-writing campaign to the state department of mental health. "We want you to be appointed the new superintendent," she said.

32

[1]

After Zelda attacked her, Wendy cultivated a habit of purposely rattling her keys as she approached the backdoor to Wilson Cottage. She didn't want to surprise anyone on the other side of the door. She knew when she was standing near the door or sitting across the dayroom on a quiet afternoon and someone unlocked and opened the door suddenly, it could be a jarring experience.

After Zelda Glover's attack on Wendy the previous month, the sheriff had been called, and he asked Wendy if she wanted to press charges. Wendy declined. It would have meant going to court, and Wendy hated going to court.

But now the administration wanted to bring Zelda back to Wilson Cottage! "Fruck-a-duck," Wendy muttered to herself, "not as long as I've got the keys to this place, they won't."

Wilson Cottage had one of the best records for assaults. Of course, the patients were more highly functioning than in many of the other units. But though the unit may have had less than its share of assaults, it still had them.

Just a few days after Wendy returned to work after her beating by Zelda, a particularly nervous patient, Robert Bullman, had assaulted a psych tech. Robert had been having a mild argument with another patient. Everything was well within the bounds of a normal disagreement until there was a blast of air as the door opened and the psych tech appeared. Before anyone knew what was happening, the patient took a wild swing at the psych tech and connected on his shoulder.

Robert, who had merely been startled, was not normally assaultive. He immediately apologized. Wendy had taken him into a seclusion room for a heart-to-heart talk. She knew he was just nervous about leaving the hospital, which he had been scheduled to do in a few days.

The attack on the psych tech would have to be reported—that was the rule—regardless of how little actual harm was done. Wendy had taken Robert into the seclusion room because he was still agitated. She knew he wasn't violent, that he was just afraid someone would want to harm him now, or that they might not let him go.

"It's okay, Robert." Wendy tried to calm him down.

"I did a bad, bad thing," he kept saying. "They're not gonna let me outta here, now. I'll never see my mom before she dies."

Wendy knew he wasn't normally assaultive, and that his agitation was out of guilt and fear rather than anger. But she also knew that if she didn't calm him down his emotions could whip into a potentially dangerous froth. She'd seen scared patients do almost as much damage to themselves and others as the psychopaths and the manic patients did on their crazy-mean binges.

"You know you shouldn't have hit Bill. But you know that and you apologized. I just want you to calm down so you can go back out there and make up with him. Okay?"

"He scared me when he came in the door like that. I thought it was the Angel of Death. I've seen the Angel of Death walking around here, so I know."

This was a man the hospital was planning to discharge in a few days.

"But you know it was Bill, right? You just got scared. We know that."

"Of course it was Bill. He just scared me. I don't want to hurt Bill. Bill's my friend. He gives me cigarettes."

Within ten minutes she had calmed Robert down and he went out and shook hands with the psych tech.

"Buddies again," Bill said.

The report would say that the assault was minor and that no special action needed to be taken with regard to the patient.

Wendy had learned early that you don't make any sudden movements around patients, no matter how sedate they appeared to be. You just always moved as calmly and deliberately as possible. The deliberate part was necessary so that the ones who were always looking at you would understand that you were in control. Once you looked confused, some of these patients would make the most of it, especially the game-players.

Which is what Zelda was. When she ran out of games, she just decided Wendy was the cause of all her troubles.

Robert Bullman was not a game-player. Oh, he tried to be. He tried to keep up with Zelda and some of the other borderline personalities. But Robert just didn't have the brains to play games very well. There are many frontiers for the damaged mind to wander. Some of the borders are with the conscienceless conniving of sociopathy, some with the smashed persona of schizophrenia. Robert's tangled borders were with a kind of mental vacancy. Everything in him was a pose, a set of superficial motions he learned from watching the others and from characters on TV. If you followed Robert four or five sentences into anything, you found the Angel of Death, a cartoon character, or some other hallucination. If you followed him a little further you found a void.

Wendy knew all about "treatment by bus ticket" and "dumping" patients. A friend who had been on grounds patrol told her that some patients had been "escorted" to the state line in the middle of the night and dropped off. This sort of thing had stopped when Dr. Greco came aboard, he said, because Greco knew and kept track of every patient in the hospital. But he was the first one in a long time to do that.

But neither Greco nor anyone else could stop the "treatment by bus ticket," because it was a matter of state and county policy, not hospital policy. When the state or county wanted a patient discharged, that patient was discharged. It was not a matter of medicine, but of money. Wendy knew it cost thousands of dollars a week to keep a patient at Bedloe, and the counties didn't like to see that money leaving their domain.

So Robert Bullman and many more like him were pronounced "stabilized" or whatever term the county officials and doctors agreed upon to mean that he or she could be discharged. A social worker would write out instructions on a small piece of paper, complete with the address and phone number of the community mental health center that would be waiting for the patient to show up promptly the next day. Along with that the patient would be given maybe a two-week supply of meds and a little paper envelope with the exact change for the bus ticket, with the destination written on the envelope. No records or charts, identification, or return address.

Robert Bullman had one of these envelopes on the day Wendy had driven him to the bus station. "This is more than most patients get, Robert," she told him. "Most of you guys just get walked to the city bus stop outside the hospital. But I had some time today. . . ." Wendy's voice trailed off into a frown as she saw Robert empty his bottle of meds out the hospital-car window. She felt a hard ball sink through her stomach.

Robert had an envelope with exactly $12.80 in it, and the name of his home city on it.

"This oughta get me to California," he said proudly.

"I don't think so, Robert," Wendy had said. "I don't think it's nearly enough to get you that far."

"My momma's there."

"Sure, Robert. Sure."

Robert had a slip of paper that had the address of the community mental health center neatly printed on it. As the car neared the bus station and slowed in the clogged traffic, he started to squirm in his seat.

"I'm going to find a place to park this car and go on in with you Robert. I want to make sure they get you on the right bus."

"I'll be okay, Wendy. I'll get to California."

There were no parking spaces. The normally three-lane street was reduced to one lane in some places by cars double- and triple-parked. Wendy circled the block once, an ordeal that took fifteen minutes—but she felt she had to go in with Robert.

He pulled the slip of paper with the address and phone number on it out of his pocket and inspected it.

"What're you doing with that, Robert?"

Robert ignored her and slipped it back into his pocket.

"I'll just get out," he said.

"No! Robert! The car is moving!"

Robert took his hands off the door handle and looked at the slow-moving traffic with a frown. He took the slip of paper out of his pocket again and put the corner between his lips.

They were at an intersection, waiting for a chance to turn onto a one-way street where traffic was moving relatively faster.

Suddenly, at the same moment that an opening cleared, Robert yanked open the car door and jumped out. Wendy yelled for him to stop, slammed the gear shift into "park" and jumped out after him. In the last glimpse she had of him as he disappeared into the crowd, he was rolling up the piece of paper with the address and phone number on it and throwing it away.

Horns blared mercilessly behind Wendy's car. She got back in, drove it to an expensive parking lot three blocks away, and ran back to look for Robert. After an hour she gave up. All the way back to the hospital she told herself that she had already done more than any other tech would have done.

But that wasn't enough, Wendy felt, and she kept whispering the knowledge to herself, giving it sharp nails to claw at the inside of her skin. Her back started twinging again, first time in months, and all the rest of that day she found herself coming up short with the patients. Not often, but often enough, she would yell at one of them for a minor offense. She even shouted in anger at little Lily Speere. The poor girl seemed to radiate vulnerability. It wasn't her mind that seemed weak, Wendy thought, it was her body, as if the delicate life in her flesh was closer to the surface.

Wendy couldn't even remember why she had scolded Lily. The girl had just turned away with a look of silent pain, and Wendy felt immediately guilty.

But that didn't stop her from angry outbursts at two other patients that same shift.

Nor did it seem to make a difference when a patient came up to her and asked her to read a bedtime story. "Are you kidding?" Wendy had barked. On her way out that night, another patient had caught up with her and asked what kind of muffins she was bringing for breakfast the next day. Wendy had just smiled a tight little crimp and said she had no idea. And there were no muffins the next morning, nor any for the next two days either. Finally, she went to the grocery store on the way home from work and bought some day-old muffins, which she threw out the truck window on her way down to the hospital the next morning.

[3]

"Am I mentally ill?" Wendy asked the psychologist, feeling a little foolish at the same time. Fruck-a-duck, she said to herself, I'm surrounded by shrinks all the damn day and here I am paying good money to talk to one. What would Doc say?

"I don't know. What makes you ask that question?" Jean Fitzsimmons, Ph.D., asked.

"Well . . . I don't know. I'm real confused. There are bad people, but we're not all bad people. A lot of people come to the hospital and put in their time and the only thing they care about is that they get paid. We get paid twice a month. Doctors get paid once a month. I worked in other mental hospitals before I came to Bedloe, and I've heard all sorts of horrible stories. You've come to the end of the line when you come to the state hospital. That's one of the stories. And then there's the one that says all we know how to do is beat up and kill patients. And we don't. We really care. We're more caring about the patients than they are in the community. In the community mental health centers it was my impression that the patients could have anything they wanted as long as they didn't bother the doctors—all the narcotics they wanted. And here we have all the guidelines, you can only give a person so much and you're restricted as to what you can give them. In a private hospital you can give them whatever you want."

"You're rambling, Wendy."

"I am. I am. I was standing next to a person who was telling me that state hospitals are so awful, that all we do is drug 'em, beat 'em up, and kill 'em. I guess I feel like we have a lot of pitfalls, and the hospital could be better, but I think that basically we all care. Well, there are a lot of us—not all of us—who do care about patients."

"Wendy, it sounds to me that when you say bad, what you mean is people who are burnt out, or who don't care. It doesn't sound like you're saying there are people who are sadistic or hurtful. But there are people who don't care. Am I right?"

"There are bad people, too."

"Tell me about them."

"I don't know. All I know is I'm taking care of one, two, three people right now who are trying to kill themselves. Those are the ones I know about. Who knows?"

"You're rambling again, Wendy."

"One of them likes to put things in his mouth. Pencils. Broken glass. He has to be watched constantly."

"I want to hear about the bad people, Wendy."

Wendy took a deep, distant breath. "This week I worked two sixteen-hour shifts. A couple of weeks ago I worked three, back to back."

"Wendy," Dr. Fitzsimmons interrupted, "I really want to hear about the bad people, and everything else. But it will have to wait until our next session."

"We did well for a first session, Wendy," the therapist said as she escorted Wendy out the door.

Standing in the street, Wendy had felt drained and her back was starting to feel tight and sore. She tried to trace back through her mind the steps that had led her to this moment, this location on the planet, but she could not. She had wanted to talk about Dan Billings and about Bert. She had wanted to talk about her mother, and about Robert Bullman and his mother. And she had wanted to make another appointment, yet she had walked right past the receptionist, whose attention had been diverted by an error in her typing.

[4]

Now, as Wendy jingled her keys, she felt like she was starting all over again. Dan said she should go to nursing school. That would be starting all over again with a vengeance. But it would be like starting all over again and working so hard just to get back to where she had been years ago. "Just to let me work with the patients the way I did when I started? Seems crazy to me."

"Life's crazy," Dan had said. "You do what you have to, Wendy."
He was annoyed at her, she could tell. "Damn, you know it'd be
more than that. You know it."

That was it. Wendy didn't know what was important anymore.
Nothing she could think of or remember or see or feel or imagine
seemed important.

But making noise with the keys and entering carefully was important, and she did that. The unit was quiet. No one met her.

At least the lights were on. Well, it got dark sooner and light later
now, so the lights were on before the staff came back from their
break and woke up the patients. Someone should be in the nursing
station, though. Unless they were called away or distracted by an
emergency or in the bathroom.

Wendy heard a shuffling and stopped dead to look around and
get a sense of where the noise was coming from. Everything was
still.

She heard bedsprings. Then more shuffling. Then the stillness
again.

Then she heard the springs groan, and a thud, and a creaking that
spread across the ceiling. As the noise passed over Wendy's head it
reached down her back like an icy transfusion, because now Wendy
knew what was happening.

She yelled for help and whirled around and ran toward the
women's dormitory. There was something blocking the door, but
the cold terror in Wendy gave her a strength she'd never had
before, and she pushed her shoulder against the door and the iron
legs of the bed screamed across the floor as the door opened.

Wendy yelled for help again when she saw the white form
wriggling on the end of the white rope, the ghost of a huge fish
struggling at the border between life and death. Lily Speere was
hanging herself. Wendy scrambled over the bed and lifted Lily by
the ankles with all the strength she had left, stretching and pushing
until the rope made of sheets went slack and the spasms stopped.
Wendy started to sob with the exertion, and then tears came from
somewhere else when she heard Lily's guttural sobs and felt quickening in the girl's bare white legs.

Women sat up in bed. A few stood up sleepily. Some were
sobbing, some looked on the scene with fascination and curiosity.
Some went for help. Between gasps for air and shouts for help,

Wendy heard a man's footsteps behind her. At last. She felt her back tiring and her shoulders cracking.

"Help me," Wendy cried. "I think she's okay. Think I got her in time."

"Somebody stole my head."

Wendy turned around just enough to see Bennett Ackerman standing naked, with folded arms. His cowboy hat was nowhere in sight.

"Get help, Bennett, please!"

"Somebody stole my head."

Lily Speere jerked twice and choked out a cough.

33

[1]

October was Doc's favorite month. There was enough warmth left for the hardier flowers, but it was a gentle warmth, and he welcomed the full, bright sun on his face. The committee's visit left a bad taste in Doc's mouth, although he was glad about the outcome. "I'm just happy it's over," he said to Alex, "because now we can all get back to work."

Work was why Doc was in Alex's office. He didn't even sit down, but paced back and forth along the far wall. He stopped in front of one of Alex's paintings. A group of men in dark coats stood solemnly on a beach and watched while three men in white, billowy clothes worked a large wooden contraption that extended a long arm out over the surf. At the end of the arm there was a chair, and strapped in the chair was a young woman screaming in drenched agony. Her thin clothes and long hair were soaked and the white fingers of the surf splashed up toward her.

"You know, Alex," Doc said, "a hundred years from now, some

260

smart-ass psychiatrist is going to have a painting of you and me doing what we're going to do today to that young woman."

Alex said, "There are already people who paint us that way."

Doc chuckled, "The funny thing is that dunking worked, too. Not as well as ECT, but it helped a lot. Manic patients. Depressed patients. It's a mystery."

"We are manipulators of mysteries, Doc. That's all there is to it."

"I'm supposed to say that, not you, Alex. You want everything to be neat and scientific. Predictable."

"Mostly, I want things to work. Is the patient prepped?"

"Rosey and Wendy are with her now."

[2]

After Lily's suicide attempt, Doc had gone to Alex and said he wanted to try ECT right away. "Sure, we can try every antidepressant made and maybe one of them will work before she succeeds in killing herself. Or maybe they'll keep her alive long enough for her to settle down on her own. In the meantime, you and I know that the longer she spends in this place the worse it is for her. This kid has a chance. Now, anyway. In six months, I wouldn't bet pocket change."

"Will the conservator go along?" Alex asked

"You mean her mother?"

"Her mother's the conservator?"

Doc smiled. "I guess even the great Alex Greco lets something in a patient's file slip every now and then."

[3]

Lily Speere's father had been a distant, stern man who was comfortable communicating with his daughter through either commands or other people's poetry. He tended to dominate his wife, who had been a promising young poet when he noticed her in one of his graduate literature classes.

In his will, Speere addressed his wife more directly and warmly than he had in years: "My dearest Sylvia, I hope now you will be able to rediscover the poetry in your own life, now that you no longer are needed to provide it for mine." Whether or not she would ever write poetry again was yet to be resolved, for Professor Speere had left little in the way of life insurance or savings.

Nevertheless, by chance, his health insurance did provide up to a year of benefits for mental illness. Although the benefits weren't enough for a private hospital, when Lily attempted suicide at least she did not have to become a ward of the state in order to obtain treatment.

Alex and Doc found Sylvia Speere a nervous, frail-seeming woman. Having seen Alex only once, when Lily had first come to the Receiving Unit, and Doc almost never, since she usually visited Lily on weekends, when Doc was off, Lily's mother did not at first know who these two men were. When they identified themselves at the blue door of the ivy-covered brick house, she first assumed that because they were doctors from Bedloe that "something terrible had happened." For a moment Alex thought she was going to faint, despite their reassurance that Lily was not hurt.

"We've gone outside channels, Mrs. Speere, because we think Lily's case warrants it. If we were to do this the way it's usually done, it could take months. We want to do something for Lily now," Alex explained.

"Lily's depressed," Doc said. "I don't think she really wants to kill herself, but she's really stuck in it right now. But I think I know what will help. I've seen this thing before in young women, and I've seen it cleared up, too."

Doc was angling for a question, but Mrs. Speere was silent, waiting for him to finish.

"Well, Mrs. Speere, I think what will help Lily is a short course of ECT. Electroconvulsive therapy."

Mrs. Speere frowned. She squeezed her hands together in a tight ball. "I thought that was considered barbaric," she said.

Alex looked at Doc, but the older man did not take his eyes off Mrs. Speere.

"Some people sincerely believe that it is, Ma'am," Doc said gravely. "But we believe it can save your daughter's life."

For her part, Mrs. Speere did not take her eyes off Doc's. There was a motherly fierceness in her, suddenly, a determination and a diligence. She said, drawing breath from some deep reserve within her, "Then what are you waiting for, doctors?"

[4]

Speaking out loud could sometimes be very difficult for Lily. She stammered and stuttered and had to fight against her anxiety and depression to get the words out. Although Doc tried to wean her of the habit in therapy, she often expressed herself by writing quick notes on a little pad.

Lily had questions about the treatment, and Doc, realizing her courage in even asking the questions in the first place, allowed her to carry out her half of the conversation on paper.

"Will it hurt?" she wrote.

Doc shook his head. "You'll be asleep."

"How will you put me to sleep?" she scribbled.

"Give you a shot. Dr. Konopski and Dr. Greco will be there, too, to help."

"Tell me exactly what you're going to do," she wrote with a frown.

"Well, we'll wheel you in to the ECT room. We'll give you the anesthetic and you'll fall asleep in a minute or so. We'll give you a muscle relaxant, too."

"W-w-why?" Lily spat, waving the pad and pencil.

"Well," Doc said, "the ECT causes convulsions. Without the muscle relaxant, the convulsions can be quite violent and you might hurt yourself."

"Gross," Lily moaned.

"Then what?" she wrote, looking into a vacancy between Doc and the green iron chair she was sitting on.

"Well, then I'll put the electrodes on your temples. When I switch the machine on, a small electric current will pass between the electrodes. And—"

"A big space helmet kind of thing?" she wrote.

"No, actually it looks more like a set of stereo earphones."

"I'll bet. Then what?"

"Well, the current's only on for a short time."

"Am I going to foam at the mouth and stuff?"

Doc shook his head. "No, Lily, nothing like that."

"My eyes will bug out?" she wrote.

Doc kept shaking his head.

"Am I gonna crap in my pants?"

"You better not! We're gonna starve you the night before."

"What, then? Will I just lie there!"

"Well, you'll twitch a bit. Like when you go to sleep sometimes. Only it will last longer."

"Gross!" she said clearly.

"You'll start to wake up a little while later."

She went back to the pad. "Will I dream?"

Doc looked at Lily, into her blue eyes, which were looking directly at him for the first time. He shook his head. "I don't know, dear. I don't know. Maybe. Let me know, okay?"

She wrote, "Will I remember my mother and father?"

Doc nodded. "Yes you will. You might be confused a bit for a while."

"Will I remember who I am?"

"Yes, Lily, you'll forget the treatment but you will remember who you are."

Lily looked away, into the vacancy again, and dropped the pad and pencil. "Then h-h-how's th-this g-g-g-gonna help at all?" she stammered.

Doc rubbed his chin. A breeze outside the window rustled the branches of the maple and a ribbon of red and yellow leaves swirled against the screen. "We don't know exactly how it helps, Lily. But I know it will help."

Lily took a deep breath, still searching the empty space, then said, "C-c-can W-wendy b-be there?"

Doc nodded.

[5]

Wendy was there, and so was Rosey, who tore himself away from his metaphysical conversations with the rapidly burgeoning Ethel Flynn long enough to attend his first ECT. They met Alex in the hall at seven that morning. George Konopski was a few minutes late, having felt a wave of nausea catch up with him as he entered the hospital. They all gathered around Doc, who had been with Lily since dawn. When Lily closed her eyes under the anesthetic, Doc remembered the last question she had written on her pad, "If you make the demons go away, will I still be able to write poetry?"

"Young woman," Doc said, taking her cold, nervous hand gently in his, "I have no intention of making the demons go away. I could not if I wanted to. The demons will still be around, Lily. If we're lucky, however, and the magic works, then we'll chase them out of you and into the world where they belong. Then you can come to terms with them face to face. They'll try to get back in, but, again, if we're lucky, you'll get a look at them outside of you and see that they are not you, that you are good and can fight them, even if they manage to creep back in. We're giving you a fighting chance, Lily. That's all. If you want to make poetry out of that, no reason why you can't."

There was a kind of solemnity to the procedure. Only words that had to be spoken broke the quiet purpose of the ritual, the movement of hands over Lily, the concentration of eyes on the simple instruments. When the current was switched on, Doc watched for the trembling and unconsciously repeated a silent wish to himself that the therapy would work, that it would burn out the devils threatening Lily's life from the inside. He had muttered this same wish every time he performed this procedure, and in fact, every time he had administered a drug or entered into an analysis. It had the quality of a prayer, he knew.

"I've never been able to split the psychological from the biological," Doc had said to Alex once. "Thought begins with a tropic reaction, like in biology class when you have an amoeba swimming around in a saline solution in a petri dish and you squirt a little hydrochloric acid, and the one-celled microscopic beast in the dish cowers in a corner as far from the spreading drop of acid as possible. That cowering has the quality of thought. Early thought is quite physical. And I suppose by simple extrapolation, the spiritual is mixed up in this, too. If we send a bolt of lightning through the temple of the spirit, if it doesn't scare the beasts into a corner, it must at least wake up the angels."

"Let's hope it doesn't singe their wings," Alex had quipped.

Doc remembered his earlier conversation with Lily. This child was an angel, and always would be. There was a quality of innocence and vulnerability that radiated from her and, Doc felt, would radiate from her no matter how much she saw in her life, no matter how worldly-wise and strong she might become. She was worried about her poetry. "Make poetry of your life," he wanted to tell her, as the words became part of his wish.

As the twitching spread across Lily's body, Rose, whose eyes were uncomfortably wide from the first moment, excused himself and could be heard retching into the toilet in the little lavatory next to the ECT room.

[6]

One night a week later, after Lily's fourth ECT session, Doc sat on a bench in a grove of trees near the parking lot and wondered where memories went and why. Lily had slept for a longer than usual length of time. That was not a problem, nor was the fact that she forgot everything about the treatments. She was confused—also expected—and the slight stammer in her speech seemed to have become accentuated. Doc wondered what wisdom of the mind or spirit sent some memories into a vault and kept them there. Perhaps the lightning bolt through the temple exposed horrors too terrible to remember. Or perhaps some simple biochemical circuits were shorted and fuses blown.

As he had after the first three treatments, Doc stayed with Lily in the recovery room and then, when she had been brought to the infirmary, had breakfast with her and stayed as long as he could before his responsibilities on the unit called him back. During the day Doc arranged for Alex, Wendy, and Rosey to visit her. After the remainder of his shift at Wilson Cottage, he had gone back to the infirmary and sat by her bed and read poetry to her for an hour, eaten dinner, and just sat.

Doc took a chocolate bar out of his coat pocket and while unwrapping it remembered his first wife. She had wanted children but had consented to holding off for a few years until Doc's practice was more established. Then, when that time came, they had been unable to conceive. She blamed Doc's drinking and left. The drinking, which had been manageable as far as Doc was concerned, went wild after that. Doc started shaving hours off his daily workload so he could start "relaxing" sooner. Then he found he could have a few cocktails at lunch and add those hours back and it made very little difference in his performance. He was calm and steady no matter what psychic storms his skills called forth from his patients, and they loved him for it.

His second wife, Milly, wanted children, too. During the first three years of their courtship and marriage, she was able to pursuade Doc not to drink. They had a son, Woodrow Jr. and for almost 20 years after that Doc was able to keep his drinking to a politely sociable minimum. When Woody was killed in Vietnam, Doc predictably fell back into a heavier drinking pattern, and Milly did not have the will to hold him back anymore.

One evening a few years later, a colleague took Doc aside and calmly said that he believed Doc was the best psychiatrist he'd ever seen, but that if he didn't stop drinking, he would personally report him to the medical quality board. Faced with the simple choice of giving up alcohol or giving up psychiatry, Doc never drank again.

Now Doc remembered the young blond woman his son brought home during the last year of his life. She had that same vulnerability as Lily, that quality of appearing to see much and yet retaining a childlike openness to life despite her extreme sensitivity. In the years after his son died, Doc often thought of this young woman and wept for her.

There was a rustling of leaves behind Doc and he turned back toward the collection of shadows that were the main buildings of the hospital.

Lily would need at least two more ECT treatments. After that, there was no telling now. Some patients were better after six and didn't need another course for many months or years, if ever. Doc couldn't tell, though he'd spent about seven or eight hours with her. He didn't expect her to sit up and sing. She had seemed more distant, and for hours had lain silent like a hurt animal. Adolescents sometimes reacted that way. Tomorrow would be a better day.

There were two ways back to his car. Doc could go through the hospital, but that would mean he might get pulled back into the unit and he was too exhausted for that. It was a longer walk around the building, but it was dark and no one would see him. He'd taken that path many times, through a grove of trees, past a grubby tangle of bushes near the far corner of the main building, and then between two sides of smaller buildings that had no windows on their facing walls.

Doc got up and stretched his arms out high over his head to loosen his back. He saw the candy wrapper on the bench and reached over to collect it. The moon was bright, but there were black clouds with white silk borders floating across the sky. This late, the hospital was relatively quiet, so when Doc passed the grove and stepped on to the gravel path between the remote corners of the buildings, the scraping of his feet echoed. He heard a rustling and then a clunk up ahead that sent a brief shiver of cold up his back. He would have lit a cigarette, but the wind was steady enough to make it impossible, so he just walked faster.

Doc heard the grunt and in an instant knew what was happening and threw up his arms in front of his face. But the first blow struck him in the belly and it felt like a baseball bat, and then there was another blow on his back. Doc knew there were two of them as he tried to cry out before they found his face, but he managed only a whimper cut short by the pain draining the air out of his chest.

They were in front of him, kicking and blocking him into the wall and trying to get him to fall. They found his face with their fists, and it felt like a hammer striking a sharp, explosive minor chord against the taut wires of his brain. Then they found his face and chest with their shoes as Doc fell.

There was a shout, then Doc saw a third form, a loud bellowing blur charging in, wearing a red cowboy hat. Doc took advantage of the momentary lull to retreat, and packed up his bio-psycho-social-spiritual bags and went into the dark recess in his mind where the memory of this would rest forever.

34

[1]

When Doc was a young man one of his best friends was a pharmacologist named Schwartz, who knew everyone and everything in the drug business. Long before any drug became public knowledge, Tolly Schwartz not only knew about it, but had samples. Schwartz had access to drugs even before their relative legality or illegality was established. He had them when they were simply "substances," or "research curiosities."

So Doc had the opportunity to find out about these substances before most people knew about them, sometimes even before they had names attached to them and were just known by research numbers. Schwartz also encouraged him to sample the more interesting varieties of "research curiosity."

These "research soirees," as Schwartz liked to call them, usually took place before or after a social evening in which Doc and his wife would visit the Schwartzes. Just before dinner Doc and Schwartz would leave the wives in the kitchen and slink out to the garage, which had not had a car in it for at least a decade. After Schwartz and his wife moved in, the garage had been rebuilt as a laboratory. Though it had a full complement of glass tubes and bottles and other chemistry what-not, the carpeted room was little more than a retreat for Schwartz, who kept enough chemicals around to give the place the comforting smell of a real lab.

Doc and Schwartz would take the drug, if the effect was pleasurable or interesting, or, as in the case of therapeutic agents meant for severe illness, watch research film clips of patients given the drug. By the time dinner was ready, Doc and Schwartz were usually able to control their faces and speech enough to hide their mental state from their wives.

But there was one weekend in the 1950s when Schwartz conspired with Doc to get together when their wives were both out of town. "We're going to need lots of time for this one," he told Doc with a kind of solemn excitement, "and we're going to need the whole house."

"What is it?" Doc asked, examining the little vial with sugary crystals in it.

"Lysergic acid diethylamide. It's called LSD, Ben."

"Hmmm. What does it do?"

Schwartz took a deep breath and let it out slowly. Doc knew he took great pleasure in these explanations. "Well, imagine your mind is an artist's studio. You know, paints and brushes and canvases. There's a truckload of paint in a universe of colors, brushes as thick as a polar bear's fur, and canvases as wide as the sky. And an artist with the creativity and manic energy of all the great masters rolled into one.

"But normally all this is tethered, limited by the boundaries inside the brain. The lids on the paint are narrow, so only tiny brushes can be dipped in. The canvases are tiny, too. Normally, the artist—the senses—uses small brushes and dips them into the paints only very carefully as he represents the world to us. As for the inner world, well, we get that only in dreams. But we're using only the surface of the brain. When you consider the exploding universe of sensation going on inside and out, the artist pretty much minds his business, wears blinders on his eyes and chains around his arms and legs. This drug takes those chains and blinders off, tears the lids off the jars of paint and blows the lock off the basement door where

the big cans of paint and the big brushes and canvases are. It
spills the paint and rips the roof off the studio, too. Sets the artist
free."

"Doctor Schwartz, could you give me a more professional explanation?"

"I'll try," Schwartz said. "Biochemically, the traffic signals and
speed limits on the neuronal pathways are obliterated. All the roads
that were closed are opened. Everything becomes a road. At the
speeds the thought and sensation impulses travel, once fueled by
this stuff, everywhere is anywhere. Imagination, memory, and sensation are all the same."

"Sounds like psychosis to me. There's a lot more than bigger cans
of paint in that basement, you know. And that artist fellow has the
eyes of a snake and the teeth of a shark."

"Well, you're right, Ben. A lot of the research on this stuff was
done by the army and is classified. But, yes, it can not only mimic
psychosis, but it can bring it on. There have been suicides, too."

Doc's eyes narrowed at his friend.

"But it's more than psychosis," Schwartz said before Doc could
gather his thoughts into a sentence. "The beauty of this drug is that
it shows us that the boundaries between sanity and psychosis are
physical and flexible. Most important, they're changeable. They
weren't erected by parents or spirits, but by chemistry and biology."

"You sending me over the border tonight, Tolly?"

"You'll be okay, I know, Ben. I'll stay with you to make sure you
don't try to fly off the roof. It's been known to happen."

"You won't take it, too?"

"No. It's usually done that way, with a sitter."

[2]

Two hours later, Doc was calmly explaining to a greatly amused
and genuinely curious Schwartz how it felt to have your male
genitals slowly disappear and be slowly replaced by a complete set
of female sexual apparatus. "I know enough about Jungian theory to
tell you that's your anima coming out and replacing your animus,
Ben," his sitter intoned solemnly.

"This is a very interesting pharmacological experiment," Doc
kept repeating, both out loud and to himself. "Do you have any idea

of the rich jungle of life that goes on in your living-room carpet?" he said, pointing down at the floor.

At one point later in the afternoon, Doc accurately described every color of paint that had ever been used on every wall of the house, claiming he could see beneath each successive layer to the color below. When he tried to tell Schwartz the colors that were yet to be painted on the wall, the pharmacologist refused to listen.

Doc insisted, but his sitter was saved by the doorbell. Doc was up and on his way to the door, and had the door open before Schwartz could stop him. It was the mailman with a special-delivery letter.

"Oh, yes, I'll be glad to sign for Dr. Schwartz. Nice day, isn't it?" Doc said. With the door closed and the mailman on his way and Doc handing him the letter, it was, for a moment, Schwartz's turn to narrow his gaze. "That mailman is a nice fellow," Doc said. "Here's your letter."

Schwartz was just about to award Doc the Pharmacological Academy Award for Best Performance in a Phony Hallucinogenic Experience when he saw the real sweat pouring out of Doc's skin.

"Gotta go bathroom fast, 'scuse me," Doc said.

Schwartz followed his friend to the bathroom, but Doc was faster. He heard Doc moaning, "Beautiful!" as he came around the corner in the hall.

Doc was standing at the vanity, eyes open as wide as eyes could get without falling out.

Doc saw the beautiful red of his blood and the hot pink of his flesh as the layers peeled away before his eyes, right down to the clean gray bone. His face, and then his whole body had melted before his eyes. Soon he didn't need the mirror anymore, he could look down at himself and see and feel his flesh come apart in delicate layers of color like a multicolored rose.

After his body had dissolved, there was nothing left, no boundary between him and what before had been not-him. There was no not-him. Doc sat at a table and part of him was the table and part of him was the chair. And all of him was the air, the house, the trees, the sky, the galaxies. "I know what it's like to be dead, Tolly," he told Schwartz, "in a universe where there is no death."

Now, almost forty years later, Doc felt dissolved all over again. He searched with his senses for boundaries between him and everything else, and could not come up with anything not-him. All his eyes could find was white, so he gave up on sight. Taste and smell were gone, too.

He could hear a low hum, which every now and then modulated slightly higher or lower. Touch was the most curious of his senses, because he could feel the existence of the world, could feel its mass under and above and around him. But the boundaries were not there, they just were not there.

Later, there were pinches in the white expanse above him.

Later still, the pinches precipitated into corners, and there were enough corners to make a room. There was plenty around him now that was not-him, but this conviction was a foggy one, and more faith than sensation.

Doc knew there was a bed, and bandages, but as far as he could tell he had melted into them the way a spill is soaked up by a rag. Then Doc remembered how terrified he would have been during that LSD trip forty years ago if he had not known it was all artificial, all a drug affecting circuits in his brain. He had not panicked then and he would not panic now, for he knew he was in a hospital and this sensation of not knowing where his body was, exactly, was also drug-induced. Most likely garden-variety painkillers, Doc thought, as he let himself go into another long sleep.

[3]

Lily Speere was standing there, radiant and saintly, and the very first thought that flashed through Doc's brain was that she had finally succeeded in killing herself and now he was dead, too, and she had met him at the gate to eternity. Doc rejected that one. But then the next thought flashed through and it was that he was dreaming.

Doc heard Alex Greco's voice.

"This bar's open, Doc."

This was not a dream, Doc decided. Alex was really there.

And so was Wendy, who was looking at Doc and crying.

Doc wondered for an instant if he had the power of speech.

"Hiya," Alex said.

Wendy forced a "Hi, Doc," through her sobs.

Doc fell asleep.

35

[1]

November came to the Bedloe Valley with a dreary stretch of gray cold in which everyone lost all memories of a generous autumn. Such warmth and gaiety in the air must be a fantasy, their senses told them. After a week in which snow threatened but never came, the sky sealed the land in a dull, sunless jar. Even when the sun broke through, the depth and color the light gave were quickly swept away on a biting wind.

At Bedloe State Hospital the grounds crew took out their heavy socks and locked the lawn mowers away. Leaf blowers and plastic bags were prepared for action. On the wards and in the offices, windows were shut and locked, and staff counted the shopping days left until Christmas. The kitchen crew planned heavier meals and the larder was checked for flour and canned fruit.

The weather perfectly reflected the mood in Wilson Cottage. Doc's absence, and the reason for it, dulled everyone's senses. Ethel Flynn had blossomed as much as she was going to and now only

274

grew heavier as she waddled about and complained to Rosey. For his part, Rosey filled in better than Wendy expected, and took over a major portion of the responsibility for medications. Understanding how much Doc was loved and missed, the physician brought in as a replacement imposed himself on the staff and patients as little as possible. Filling Doc's shift with another psychiatrist was not enough to restore the unit, however. Because everyone moved a little slower in their confusion and depression, the most experienced staff had to be shuffled around from shift to shift. Wendy bore the heaviest burden during the early, gloomy weeks of the month. She worked double shifts twice a week and sometimes never left the hospital for almost twenty hours. On a few of these occasions she was able to take a full twenty-four hours off, but most of the time she was not gone more than eight.

Mistakes were made. Laundry was sent out twice, or not at all. Patients who needed escorts back from jobs or programs elsewhere on the grounds were stranded. An excursion to a shopping mall was forgotten by the staff until the van drove up. The entire unit was late getting ready for breakfast three days in a row.

The changes going on within the hospital were compounding Wilson Cottage's difficulties. Staff in other units were leaving, either voluntarily or otherwise, and the administration was calling on a lot of the veterans to float here and there to fill in the gaps. Because Wilson Cottage patients required a minimum of supervision, a lot of its staff was being rotated out while inexperienced people were rotated in.

When psych tech Billy Parker, a seventeen-year veteran of the hospital, showed up at Wilson Cottage late one afternoon to carry out a special assignment, there were no regular staff members on the ward. Asking too many questions would never be one of Billy Parker's problems. *Just keep calm, smile, be firm and kind to the patients, never refuse a task, keep your mouth shut and your hands off the women patients* was the advice Billy had received from an older psych tech during his first week at the hospital. These rules had served him well for seventeen years: Billy and his wife had a three-bedroom house, a motor home, and drove a new car every three years. How many of the guys who dropped out of Valley Tri-C the first year could say as much?

Billy Parker liked Wilson Cottage, especially during the day when most of the patients were at their jobs. The unit was always relatively quiet, calm, safe, and clean. Never any filth on the walls and floor like some other units he floated into every now and then. Wilson Cottage seemed to have more than its share of celebrities, too. He'd heard they'd just done a shock treatment and the word was that maybe there'd be a lobotomy there before too long. There was that psych tech, Wendy, who was supposedly going hot and heavy with a psychologist, and even a student doctor making it with one of the patients, a pregnant one, too. You could bet a whole lot of nothing would be done about that one, Billy figured.

Billy recognized the psych tech temporarily in charge at Wilson Cottage. Kate Flannery was an experienced floater. She kept her units clean and quiet and didn't ask questions. She knew Billy always got his orders straight. Billy didn't like to run this procedure with an unknown, because then you had to explain what you were doing and, if the person wasn't hip, they wanted to see more paperwork than you had.

"I've got a discharge for the five-thirty bus, Kate."

The next day, when the mistake was discovered, Wendy had to be physically restrained by Rosey from attacking Kate Flannery and verbally restrained by her union rep from filing charges against both Billy and Kate. "They're brother techs, Wendy, and they were just following orders," the rep pleaded.

The orders Kate and Billy were following had come through the hospital accounting department. Apparently, funds for this patient's care had been cut off. The insurance company had suddenly withdrawn payment. Since the bureaucracy had no official term for "sudden discharge to protect the quarterly profits of the insurance company," the paperwork went down as "scheduled discharge." No one was present on the ward who knew this patient well enough to know that she was not scheduled for discharge. So when Wendy came in the next day with a fresh box of muffins and found that Lily Speere had been driven to the bus station and dropped off the night before, Rosey had to be torn away from therapy with Ethel Flynn long enough to give the psych tech a mild tranquilizer before she broke something.

[2]

Lily thought that maybe the man who came to get her would take her to see Doc. Wendy had promised she would take her, but said they should wait until a day or two after her next ECT.

"Now, some techs will just drop you off, but I'll take you in and get your ticket for you," the man said when he parked the car on the busy city street.

Lily started to feel scared when he took her by the arm and walked her into the bus station. Some of the people sitting on the concrete steps and low parts of the wall looked like the people at the hospital. Only they were dirtier, their clothes darker, and their eyes were red and scary. An old feeling stated to creep into Lily, first into her memory, and then it tightened its fingers in a band around her throat.

"D-d-d-d-doc?" she managed to say as she slowed down.

Billy was looking around in the smoky air of the bus station when he felt the tug on his arm. "Huh? C'mon, you're goin' home, now."

"H-h-h-huh?" Lily stammered. She scolded herself inside because she couldn't talk to this man the way she talked to Doc or Wendy. She had plenty to tell him, too, but the words just got all crowded inside. He wouldn't understand, not any of her poetry or what she was feeling now. No one would understand her poetry.

He tugged on her arm and she jerked ahead a step or two, then fell back into step with him.

"You should be happy to get out of that place, girl!" Billy said.

Lily wanted to spit the foaming words out of her mouth, but the foul air of the terminal pressed in on her and she started to feel dizzy. People were looking at her and frowning and she thought maybe something was wrong with her clothing or her hair was messy. She spent ten minutes combing her blond hair every morning, just the way Wendy taught her. "So much silk, so much beautiful silk!" Wendy called Lily's hair.

When Billy was at the counter buying her ticket, the clerk looked kind. Maybe she would listen. Lily tried to pick out just the right words, the simple ones, but all that came out was "Muh-muh-muh-muh-staaaake!"

The clerk ignored her and released a quick, tight smile at Billy.

As they walked away from the counter, Billy stopped short and cursed. "I forgot to put a quarter in the goddamn meter and there's a damn cop writing tickets!" He started to bolt toward the car, searching for change in his jeans, then he stopped short and cursed again. "Goddamn the state! I don't have any change!" He looked at Lily, panic and anger in his eyes. She stared at him for a moment, and then nodded and started fumbling in her purse.

"Jesus, what am I doing accepting money from a patient?" Billy spat.

Suddenly Billy pulled Lily's hand out of her purse and thrust the ticket into it. "Take this. Your bus is right over there—Jesus, I can't afford no parking ticket in this town!—you'll be okay. You're going home, that's all!"

"Muh-muh-muh-!" Lily choked, but Billy ran away and didn't turn around. Lily started to chase him but a crowd of boys pushed through the glass doors and blocked the way. Lily felt their eyes on her and when they were past she saw the hospital car speeding down the street past the terminal.

Lily felt her composure drain and remembered more of her fear as the empty space was created within her. Doc and Wendy had forgotten about her. *Nobody cared about Lily, nobody loved her. They had their own business to take care of.*

No, that wasn't true, Lily told herself.

But it didn't matter. Whatever her brain said, her heart felt heavy and sad within the frail shell her body had become.

A fat woman bumped Lily as she hurried past toward the ticket windows. Lily's purse jumped out of her hands, but the drawstring top held its contents inside. Lily picked it up and looked at her ticket before she put it inside.

The destination on the ticket was not a hometown or even a place to Lily, it was a thick vortex of pain. Her head started to spin when she heard the name repeated on the loudspeaker.

People were getting up and heading for the rear doors, which were under a sign that read ALL BUSES.

Lily closed her eyes but that made the dizziness worse. Her legs felt tired and she wished Doc were alive—No, Doc *was* alive. Wendy said he got hurt and then the young doctor came in and gave her a shot when she started crying and coughing. Doc was just hurt, but her *father* was dead. *Oh, that.* That was still true and there was nothing Lily could do about it. It would always be true. *Father would always be gone, wherever the dead go, wherever that was.*

Lily had always liked to think about that. The idea of following, of going where the dead go, sometimes had a palpable flavor that tempted an appetite in her, the way the anticipation of an ice-cream cone stimulates all the senses of a child.

Lily felt like sitting. There were people who looked just like the people at the hospital, and they were sitting vacantly on blue plastic chairs. She could sit there forever.

Then she heard the name again, and this time it sounded like there might be a reason to go there. After all, there was no bus to take her back to the hospital, even if the people there cared about her at all.

Lily felt her heart flutter as she approached the glass doors. She could see the huge buses in the lot beyond. She started through the door behind a man who hurried ahead of her and then let the door swing back into her arm. The blow knocked her purse out of her hand and this time its contents spilled on the sidewalk. Lily got down on her hands and knees and started scooping up the coins and scraps of notepaper with the beginnings of poems written on them. People hurrying through the doors to their buses barely managed to avoid her, and a few trampled over some of the papers.

Lily heard an engine roar and she lunged for the last poem as the exhaust blast from the bus blew it away. She snatched the poem in midair and stuffed it into her purse.

The door of the bus was still open. Lily ran for it and made the step in time. The door snapped shut behind her and she climbed the remaining two steps.

"Ticket, please, miss," the driver said without looking at her.

Lily opened her purse and panicked. The ticket wasn't there. She dug her hand in as far as it would go and searched for the narrow card. Nothing. Wait . . . there it was! She pulled out the ticket and handed it to the driver.

The driver grimaced, shook his head, mumbled an obscenity and handed the ticket back to Lily as he stopped the bus. "Wrong bus, miss. You'll have to get off."

The door swung open. Lily frowned. The pavement seemed liquid to her, like a deep, congealing ocean of tar. She stepped off the bus and the door slammed behind her. The bus roared off and she was standing in the middle of the narrow ramp to the street, choking sick on the soursweet smell of the diesel exhaust. A horn blared and she jumped to the side as a second bus rushed past.

After the bus was gone, Lily stared at the empty space where, just seconds before, thousands of pounds of metal had sped by. The bus driver had not seen her until the last second, Lily thought, as she started to develop a curiosity about the space.

She heard another bus coming.

Lily took a step out into the space . . . and the appetite didn't go away. She took another step, and now she could hear the big tires of the bus whining on the pavement. The appetite was not in the space, but beyond it now. She took her steps faster and bolted as the bus's horn blared and the brakes began to screech.

Lily hugged the gritty concrete wall on the far side of the ramp.

The bus released its brakes and roared past, horn blaring.

"D-d-d-damn!" she cried.

Lily crept along the wall of the ramp until she was out into the nervous air of the cramped terminal lot, where buses were jockeying for a position at the gate or clumsily backing up to get out. A bus had just backed out from its gate and was swinging around toward the ramp. Lily read the letters above the windshield and started frantically waving. Her eyes were pleading to make contact with the bus driver's and her hands were gesturing the way a child does when she's too scared to talk, arms straight up, hands bent and waving as if she were fanning away a swarm of butterflies—or, perhaps, trying to be a butterfly. Lily's eyes were all fright and pleading.

The bus swung over to her and the driver opened his window. Lily fought to form the words. She wanted this bus so desperately, and the words that would express her desire clearly could not be summoned in the foreign language of the profane world.

All of this in an instant: Her fingertips nervously danced around her face and almost came together in prayer as she tried to speak.

"I w-w-w-wan-n-n-na g-g-go h-h-home!" Lily stammered, with terror in her eyes that the driver wouldn't understand her poetry and so would abandon her. She squinted in the cold and a tear ran down her cheek. Behind her another bus roared past and the confusing, unkind swirl of the terminal started to reach for her like a storm tide.

The instant was over. The driver nodded to her and opened the door. Lily ran around and flew up into the bus. She sat down with a triumphant thump, victorious as any general. She struggled, but now it was to contain her joy.

"I'll take your ticket, miss," the driver said, smiling at her through the mirror. "When you're ready."

36

[1]

Since Walter's illness, Thanksgiving had been a rough holiday for
Fran. The few years that Walter was either living at home or able to
come home, the day was, at best, unpredictable and tense. She
always tried her best to make the day perfect, to bake the turkey just
the way Walter liked it when he was young, and to prepare all his
favorite dishes along with it. But something always happened.

One year Walter got upset and cried when Brad started carving
the turkey. Frank tried to comfort him, but Walter wailed and just
stormed out of the house, still bawling. Fran called the police, left
Brad home in case Walter returned on his own, and drove around
the streets looking for her son. He was brought home by the police
late the same night.

One year Walter seemed fine all through dinner. He even talked
energetically about the prospects for getting a job or going back to
school. But then he started rambling on about how his psychiatrist
was not listening to him when he tried to tell him what was really

282

on his mind. The rambling accelerated into a runaway locomotive of accusations, until Walter picked up the plate of turkey remnants and flung it at the wall. Then he started throwing knives and forks and plates. Fran shouted at him to please stop, but he kept on destroying the table as if he didn't hear her.

Finally, Brad screamed at the boy and Walter looked up from his destruction and glared at them both with a dark fury in his eyes. Then he ran into the bathroom, locked himself in, pulled the towel rack out of the wall, and started smashing the huge wall mirror. Fran called the police and, after they arrived, sobbed in terror that they might draw their guns as they talked their way into the bathroom and took her son back to the clinic.

The last year Walter had a Thanksgiving at home he got up from the table during dinner and just paced back and forth in the hall, mumbling to himself and seeming to carry on a conversation with people from the clinic. Fran and Brad tried to get him to go to bed, but he just shook his head and continued his marathon. They went to bed but didn't sleep, hoping Walter would calm down. Hours later, when the house was quiet, they emerged from their room and found him asleep on the floor, curled up like a dog outside their door.

The years when Walter was not at home were not much better. Fran and Brad stayed home until noon, and then called Walter at whatever facility he happened to be in at the time. Sometimes he would seem depressed, sometimes angry or peevish—never at them, usually at one of the staff or at other patients. But he always told them what he was having for Thanksgiving dinner, and Fran had to hold herself like a stone as he read the pathetic institutional menu. After the call, after all the calls from Walter, Fran would go to her room alone and sit by the window and stare at a photo of her mother as a young girl. She would wonder where the quality of mercy was in the universe.

Then Fran and Brad would steel themselves for a holiday dinner at Brad's sister's house. Elaine and her husband Jack always had a full house of relatives and in-laws at Thanksgiving, and they always called to make sure Fran and Brad were going to come. "As long as you're going to be alone on the holiday" was the way they put it. So Fran and Brad drove to the subdivision called Longshadow Hills and stopped at the entrance to tell the guard their name. He checked it against a list and then saluted and opened the gate for them to pass.

Brad always made some comment about whether the gate was to keep Elaine and her neighbors in or to keep "us riffraff" out. Fran just thought it was a strange way to live. As their car got older and older, however, she felt more and more like she had the answer to Brad's question.

Elaine and Jack's house was a sprawling ranch, a house made for parties. Elaine always asked her brother and sister-in-law about Walter when they first entered the house and were alone in the marbled foyer. She would listen attentively for a few moments, make a supportive comment or two, and give Fran a hug before escorting her into the midst of the other guests in the kitchen. The kitchen opened into a large dining room, which opened into a vast carpeted living room with leather sofas. Elaine was not one for formality, so dinner was always a loud, disorganized affair with more chatter than prayer, although Jack always thanked the Lord for "this bounty which we are about to receive."

"From the looks of it, you've already received it," one of the guests from the neighborhood always said.

[2]

This year, the plan for Fran and Brad was somewhat different. They would still spend the holiday with Elaine and Jack, but they had to leave early. The staff of D-7 had planned a special Thanksgiving open house for the patients and their relatives. To allow the staff to have the holiday itself with their families, the special dinner was planned for the day after Thanksgiving. Fran and Brad planned to leave early so they could drive up to Bedloe that night, stay in a hotel near the hospital, and be at the ward relaxed and refreshed instead of tired from a three-hour drive.

As usual, by the time turkey was on the plates, Fran had loosened up and relaxed into the merry surroundings. Brad's other brother Tom, her favorite in-law, always made sure her wine glass was full and joked with her about being the "designated drinker" at the party.

"They're raising our taxes again," Tom said when most people were done eating but the table still had the hushed murmur of a meal and had not progressed to busy chatter.

"I don't know what this country's coming to," Jack said, picking his teeth with the corner of a matchbook.

"And all these people out of work," Fran said.

The table went silent for a moment. Jack and Tom and Fran looked at each other, trying to establish a connection. Tom nodded politely. Jack grimaced. "There are plently of jobs. They just don't want to work. Like all these homeless bums."

Elaine perked up. "The other day, you know, there were two of them trying to just walk into the neighborhood. Thank God for the gate!"

"It's such a relief to live here. I know I can let my kids play in the yard now and I don't have to worry," a neighbor woman said. "I had to watch them every minute when we lived over on Thomas Street."

"These enclosed neighborhoods are a great thing," Jack said. "I don't know why more developments don't do it."

"Just about all the subdivisions out in California do it already," Tom pointed out.

"The neighborhood association over at Sunset Park got together and now they're building a wall around their subdivision. City tried to stop it, but they went to court and the city backed down."

"Of course they did. They don't want to set a legal precedent. Every neighborhood's going to do it. They know the government can't protect their property rights anymore," Tom said. "All the tax money goes for welfare."

"I don't know," Fran said. "I just wish they'd do something useful with our tax money. I mean, instead of building all those bombers and submarines . . . I know the hospital where Walter is could use more money."

The chatter at the table crashed into a muddy silence.

"Well, I guess," Tom said. "How is Walter, Franny?"

A few people got up from the table.

"Much better, thanks, Tom," Fran said. "He's been on a new medication and . . ." Tom's eyes had glanced away and were picked up and held by Jack's, and then Elaine's.

Jack waited until he was sure Fran wasn't going to continue her sentence and then said, "I'll help clear the table, girls. The football game doesn't start for half an hour yet. But next year, Elaine, let's hire a maid, okay?"

[3]

Later, as she and Brad drove out through the gate, which was
stark and floodlit in the golden light of dusk, Fran felt that she was
seeing the wall for the first time. It was made of decorative stone,
about eight feet high, and it truly went around the entire subdivision. She wondered what the country would look like once every
neighborhood was walled off.

There was a gathering weight inside her, which she could not yet
identify. She turned and looked back at the gate in time to see the
barrier, a steel fence, slide back into place. She knew then that the
weight was the heavy emptiness of loss. When Walter had been a
small boy, he loved to visit his Aunt Elaine. Fran would sometimes
drop him off in the early afternoon and he would spend the rest of
the day, and sometimes the night, too.

Elaine always kept plenty of Walter's favorite chocolate cookies in
the cookie jar, and Walter knew she did not keep a very good count
of them. And Jack was Walter's favorite uncle. Since he bought a
new car every year, Jack's cars never lost that new-car scent that
excited Walter. And all Jack's cars had electric windows, and he
would let Walter play with them no end.

It wasn't them, it wasn't them, it wasn't them, Fran kept repeating
to herself, stoking the embers of a virtue she had once called charity
but which she now just wished would give off enough faint light so
she could read her own sanity in the lines of her life. It wasn't them,
she repeated, it was a hammer or a comet or an avalanche or an
earthquake or a tornado or a hurricane or a tidal wave or a virus or
a cancer or a blind fist. It was God's will, or it was just bad luck. It
was the way things were. Her son would always be on the wrong
side of the world's walls and gates.

Fran wanted to acknowledge this loss to her husband, as if there
might be some grace in the knowledge. She wanted to say: Brad,
you know if Walter were to come here, they'd never let him past
that gate.

But Fran kept silent. The knowledge would be a burden on Brad,
whereas to Fran it was another step in her liberation, another
sharpening of the definition of her life. While Brad suffered the
losses and allowed the weight of them to drag him back into a stolid

kind of sorrow, Fran let the sorrow be a knife whose weight pushed
the blade through her life to cut away the superfluous layers of
expectation and longing. Her life was to become a warrior, and
every piece of finery that was torn away left her lean and muscled to
face the Enemy.

Fran turned her face to the window and felt the cool glass on her
forehead. The sky looked like snow, but she knew Brad could make
it through the worst snowstorm. "I miss our son," she said, finally.
"I miss him, Brad."

Brad swallowed and coughed and kept his eyes on the road
straight ahead. "I miss him, too, Franny."

37

Alex let his fingers run slowly over the letters of the brass plaque: "Built in 1913 to care for the mentally ill of the state." He tried to connect the words of three or four generations ago with the reality of today. Forged in metal, the words had a solidity. The men and women who decided to use these words must have been sincere and determined in their purpose. By touching the metal he hoped he could draw from that determination and feel the metal's strength and worthiness to be cast as a witness for history.

No, it was just a highway marker. They had to put something here, so they put this.

But the hospital was there. Alex could see it when he looked up. It had substance, too: stone and metal and wood and glass and fabric and plastic.

Winter was almost a month away, but most of the leaves were on the ground. There had been no appreciable snow yet, but the rain and wind of three brutal storms had ripped them loose from the trees. Alex looked out over the mile or so of stark forest between him and the hospital and tried to pick out a building at a time. How had things changed in the past six weeks, since Akbar's departure?

Doc had almost been killed. If the patient Bennett Ackerman hadn't been returning late from a visit to the canteen and happened by, Doc would be dead now. The men who had beaten him were not there to warn Doc, they were there to make an example or to wreak vengeance. His attackers had not been patients. Patients would not have escaped so easily.

Well, Alex mused, this was the way human beings still accomplished things. Transitions were not easy for us. Despite all the bureaucratic fineries, the hospital was a battleground and always would be. The police were "doing their best," as they had done in January rape-murder of the young patient Deborah Smith. But Alex had enough forensic experience to know that more than 95 percent of violent crimes that were solved were done so only by confession. The Bedloe county police and the state police were not good enough to win against those odds.

Alex had helped keep a vigil at Doc's bedside after the beating. Doc had awakened several times and not recognized him, or Wendy, or Rosey, or anyone.

During one of Alex's later visits, they exchanged the usual jokes and chatter, but when the room was clear of other visitors he leaned over close to Doc and told him to get an attorney.

"What the hell for?" Doc whispered.

Alex explained that he had learned that the hospital was going to approach Doc with its own attorney to pressure him to sign a waiver releasing the hospital and the state of any responsibility in his "accident." As a matter of fact, he warned, before the attorney moved in, Alex, himself, as director of the medical staff, might be asked to speak to Doc . . . in an official capacity.

"Do they think I'm going to sue?"

"Aren't you?" Alex asked.

"Actually, I haven't given it a hell of a lot of thought."

"That area of the grounds should have been well lit," Alex confided. "There are lights there. Don't tell anyone where you heard this."

"Maybe I should be grateful those lights were off. If their aim had been any better I might be dead."

"Recognize them at all?"

Doc shook his head. "They weren't patients."

"I assumed they weren't."

Doc seemed to be thinking hard about something.

"Giving some thought to my advice?" Alex asked.

Doc chuckled. "I know just the man. A good friend of mine. He'll keep them guessing, anyway."

"Who knows, you might get a settlement that would allow you to retire in style."

"Who said anything about retirement?"

"Are you coming back to the hospital?"

Doc looked away and was thinking again.

"You know, I haven't given it much thought. I guess I haven't given much of anything much thought. It seems I'll have to learn to think all over again."

As would Alex. "You'll have to learn to think like an administrator," Maria had said on one of their walks.

"I thought I already did," Alex had replied.

But he knew that he really didn't. Through his entire time at Bedloe, Alex's thinking had the style of a subversive more than anything else. With Sam in charge, Alex had fit into the role perfectly, since Sam suspected everyone of subversion and Alex certainly disagreed enough to warrant the label.

But now, what?

It was more than modesty that compelled Alex to demure when loyal staff and friends tried to push him into the superintendent's chair ahead of the state's decision. Alex initially felt a rush of power, a thrill at having won. But soon thereafter, a burdensome responsibility hurried in and hovered over him darkly. He was still working on the painting of his dream, but his progress felt slower.

The gust of wind that came up the valley promised winter, and Alex tucked his hands into his pockets. His chilled fingers found something in one pocket, a card or. . . . It was a photograph Fran Channing had asked her husband to take with their instant camera at the Thanksgiving open house at D-7. And then she had given it to Alex. The photo was only an hour or so old. In it Walter Channing was smiling proudly through his concentration while his mother beamed. And then Alex noticed something he had not seen before. Fran Channing's right hand was clenched in a fist, and the fist was held shoulder high.

"Yes, I want it," Alex muttered to himself. Then he said it clearly, out loud, into the now still, damp air hanging like a filmy membrane between him and the hospital. *"I want it."*

38

The call came on Christmas Eve day. Not only was Alex not appointed, but the new superintendent of Bedloe State Hospital would be another man with no medical training, a bureaucrat who had spent the first three years of his career as a social worker, but had removed himself further and further from direct patient involvement over the following twenty-five years.

"The successful bureaucrat never gets into a fight at all, over anything," Alex said dryly to Doc, who was out of the hospital and visiting.

"You knew what the risks were," Doc stated. With a smile on his face, to Alex's consternation. "You committed a bureaucratic mortal sin by not playing the administration's game. But you couldn't have played the game, anyway, could you?"

"I don't know. It wasn't anything I did that got rid of Akbar," Alex said. "He exposed himself. The system certainly didn't get rid of him because it's aligned with my goals."

Feeling his forehead flush, Alex tried to change the subject. "You coming back, or you just here for the party?"

"Just here for the party, today. Neither my physician nor my attorney will let me come back just yet."

"You mean you want to?" Alex asked.

Doc caught Alex's eyes and held them. "You sound bitter, Alex. Are you staying here?"

Alex swung his chair halfway around and looked out the window. "I'm not bitter. It's a relief."

"Then why all this runoff about the system not being aligned with your goals? After all the years you've been a psychiatrist, when has the system been aligned with any goals that made any sense at all? The system is aligned with money and power and paperwork, Alex."

"I'm depressed, Doc."

"You're angry, Alex. What are you angry at?"

"Our society is going into a decline. We're learning to accept a greater and greater level of brutality, not only in the behavior of those we identify as criminals, but also in ourselves. And we're believing that this is the way society was meant to be, in fact, the way it always was, and that the thrust of human evolution does not contain the responsibility to make human society more decent, more humane. Instead, if you don't have the resources to take care of yourself, then you deserve anything and everything that befalls you."

"You're really pissed off about not getting this job, aren't you."

"Okay. I am. I am."

"Alex, philosophers and assorted angry folk have been declaring the decline of Western Civilization long before I was practicing sandlot psychiatry on my neighborhood buddies. The Orient isn't exactly known for its noble aspirations these days either."

"Okay, so the whole world is in a fix. But it's more than that. Maybe I am depressed, but I'm breathing the same air we all breathe, that's why. What's wrong with us? We no longer view our society or the world as a productive organ, but as a place to compete for limited resources. We no longer believe in the expansion of life. Those who believe life is a constant competition in which someone has to lose if someone wins, are not only in the driver's seats of our politics and business and medicine, but they are also defining our moral agenda, the aspirations of our entire civilization."

Doc stared at Alex for a long minute before speaking.

Doc pointed at one of Alex's paintings, a small one that depicted three men in tricornered hats escorting a man with a cloth sack over his head through a dark forest. "When this country was in its infancy, as your painting shows, the mentally ill were often kidnapped from the town square or the jail and dropped off across the county line so they would be somebody else's problem. No different from what's going on now. You know, Alex," Doc said, "at least two of the men who signed the Declaration of Independence participated in such shenanigans. And quite of few of them, while creating a document that is still the world's model for self-government, had slaves—whom they no doubt treated a lot better than their lunatics, who were more often than not kept in cages like dogs. Progress is a funny thing. It doesn't happen in a linear fashion, with things getting better and better all the time, although we may feel more comfortable moving through a frightful history if we believe that they do. History is a dance up a mountain, not a stroll, or even a difficult climb. We do-si-do up and down, back and forth from what you call savagery—which, by the way, you should understand is never too far from the surface no matter how fancy your clothes happen to be."

Alex rubbed his forehead. "What is it about this country that wants to ignore the suffering of its weakest members?"

"Alex, you're talking about human nature, not America."

"No, I'm talking about a mass decision to turn away, to take a step back toward savagery."

"Again, Alex, if you don't want to call it human nature, call it gravity, inertia, original sin, the confounding backward current of mortality. Whatever you want to call it."

"No, Doc. Human nature, gravity, and original sin explain why our efforts are not 100 percent effective—when we try. They do not explain why we've decided not to try. I fear for my country. We're becoming a Third World country, a banana republic, medically. A third of the country already is there. We're experiencing a devil's triage, where the more severe the illness, the less care that's given. The helpless and the politically weak, or inept, are being cut off from quality medical care. The middle class is already cut off from quality care for the mentally ill. Pretty soon we'll have a two-tiered system. The rich—maybe 5 percent of us—will get quality care, everyone else will take their chances."

"You're bitter, Alex," Doc said.

"I'm angry and frightened. Terrified, if you must know."

Doc examined Alex's face for a long minute. "Alex, it goes back and forth. Okay, so we're taking some steps back now, as a society. We're also making some progress. We're setting the groundwork for what may add up to the next forward leap."

Alex realized he was pushing Doc too close, so he tried to calm down. "You came of age at the threshold of one of our steps forward."

"I did, and I expect to see the next one begin."

"Hmm. Okay. Okay, Doc. I'll salvage some hope from that, and from some other places. Science, maybe."

Doc stood up and reached across the desk to grab Alex's arm. "No, Alex. Don't patronize me. Forget science and politics and religion. Hope comes from one place, and that's the human heart, when it shares with other hearts its dreams and its pain and its refusal to give up."

39

When word reached Wendy that Robert Bullman, the patient she had dropped off at the bus station in the fall, was back in the Receiving Unit and would be transferred to Wilson Cottage by Christmas Eve, she showed no signs of surprise. "I knew he was coming back," she remarked casually. "I even bought a Christmas present for him."

In fact, Wendy had bought several more Christmas presents than she needed. The hospital provided presents for every patient, in the form of a grocery sack full of toiletries and donated clothes. "Just a lousy brown grocery bag," she spat. "Fruck-a-duck!" Her first year at the hospital, she bought red ribbons to tie on every gift bag, but the whole affair was still a pathetic excuse for Christmas as far as she was concerned. So every year after that, Wendy bought every patient in Wilson Cottage a little present, which she wrapped in the brightest Christmas paper she could afford. She tried to give each patient something he or she would really appreciate, and always bought a few extra presents, wrapped them, and brought them along to the hospital. Patients who had no relatives always got at least one extra present from Wendy, usually some specially baked and wrapped goodies, like a dozen of Wendy's chocolate chip cookies, which were legendary in Bedloe Valley and considered a controlled substance around Wilson Cottage.

Wendy also fired up her oven the week before Christmas and baked cakes, pies, muffins, and special breads. This year she had an extra set of hands in the kitchen. Dan Billings had started coming over one or two evenings a week. They would take walks in the woods, and usually wind up in Wendy's bed. But Wendy always grew restless around 10:30 or 11:00, and Dan would take this as a signal to leave. Wendy didn't stop him. When she told him about all the baking she would be doing, wondering if it would frighten him away, Dan smiled and offered to roll up his sleeves. Wendy looked at this out of the corners of her eyes, but nodded that she would have an apron ready for him.

Dan wasn't much good as a cook, Wendy found out right away. On the first night of her baking marathon, a Sunday, she had to throw out an entire batch of cookies because he left the baking soda out of the recipe. After that, she gave him only simple cleanup tasks. She was still looking sideways at him on Tuesday, about a quarter to midnight, which was when the last batch of the night usually came out of the oven. But on Wednesday night she realized that she was a full day ahead of schedule, and it was because Dan had kept the kitchen clean and orderly while she mustered flour, sugar, butter, and other ingredients into a standing army of Christmas cheer.

Dan didn't leave that night, and around three in the morning Wendy woke up because the moonlight shone in her eyes, and there was Dan, wide awake, looking at her. "You're weird," she said, and went back to sleep.

[2]

The rest of the Wilson Cottage staff took care of other preparations for the Christmas party, although Wendy was kept informed of every detail. When they brought in the decorations provided by the hospital, Wendy took one look at the faded and frayed collection and threw it right in the trash. "I wish they'd have that accreditation committee come one time at Christmas," she declared. "Then maybe we'd get some new decorations. Those scraps looked like they might go back a hundred years!" Then Wendy took up a collection for new decorations. "We'll store them here, or at home," she said. "They'll belong to the unit." Some staff members gave more than others, but everyone gave something, even a few of the patients who overheard Wendy collecting from staff.

By Christmas Eve day, Wilson Cottage was gayly tinseled and garlanded and angeled and belled. There were even battery-operated candles in all the windows, including those of the nursing station. Patients left for their jobs extracting promises from Wendy and the other staff that the party wouldn't start until they returned from work.

All promises were faithfully kept. Not until every patient was assembled was the food brought out. Since several of Wilson Cottage's patients worked in the hospital kitchen, a few of the therapists and psych techs had commandeered the kitchen for a couple of hours after dinner the day before and transformed the usual hospital-food ingredients into a true Christmas feast. Doc, who arrived with Alex Greco in time for the food, pronounced them "true alchemists."

Patients and staff gathered around Doc, and there were more than a few hugs. When Doc felt the hug to be unnecessarily delicate, he said, "You can hug tighter. If I ain't broke by this time, you're not going to break me." The staff already knew that the issue of Doc's return was not yet settled. But the patients, although advised beforehand, did not respect decorum and asked him if he was coming back anyway. Doc smiled, always touched the patient gently on the shoulder or the arm, and said, "Well, I'd like to come back. But it's up to my doctor. I've got a doctor, too, now. But he's a meaner sonofabitch than I ever was."

At 4:15, just as the line was forming at the buffet, Patty Robito's husband showed up to take her away for his conjugal visit. Wendy saw a shadow darken across Patty's face. She made her way to Patty's side before the man got to her, hugged her, and whispered something in her ear. Patty smiled meekly and then left with her husband for the nearest, cheapest motel.

Around 4:30 there was a phone call for Wendy from the Receiving Unit. Normally, they would ask that a psych tech come down to pick up a new patient. But the Receiving Unit, whose total recognition of the holiday was to tack up the dusty ornaments provided by the hospital, wanted to deliver a patient, and send three or four staff to do it. "Fruck-a-duck," Wendy said. "You only need one for Robert. He's harmless. Just gotta keep him from getting lost." Twenty minutes later, Robert Bullman, who had bolted for California, was welcomed back to Wilson Cottage. The Receiving Unit staff stayed on until the crew that had been left behind showed up to retrieve them. Wendy sent them all back with cookies and other assorted goodies.

Wendy noticed that Dorothy Weston, who normally had a voracious appetite, seemed to be only picking at her food. "Anything wrong, Dorothy?" she asked.

The young mother and attempted-murderer wiggled her head back and forth. "No. Sister has me on a diet. She says I'm getting too fat and it's a sin."

Just then Sister Matthew appeared and Dorothy seemed to shrink. "Merry Christmas, Wendy," the nun said. "Doesn't our little Dorothy look better and better?"

As the couple walked away, Wendy made a mental note to talk to Dorothy's social worker and therapist.

At 5:15 there was another phone call, this time from the infirmary. Wendy answered, but the nurse on the other end wanted to talk to Dr. Rush. Wendy said she couldn't see him in the crowd and couldn't she take the message? The nurse asked Wendy to have Doc call her as soon as possible and then hung up. Wendy did one turn around the dayroom looking for Doc, and then heard that he had left with Dr. Greco. No one knew if he'd be back.

Bennett Ackerman received his Christmas present early, a new "heavy hat," which he placed on his head with no small ceremony. He immediately lit up with a solemn, almost reverent joy. He seemed to grow several inches in height, and for the rest of the day alternated between picking at the buffet and fabricating stories of his life before the hospital. "My time in the CIA was not glamorous, no way. Why, one time in Havana. . . ." If he happened to be telling the story to a woman, he always ended it by politely asking her to dance. The carols Wendy had arranged to have piped in from the nursing station were not exactly the kind of music that set a lady's toes to tapping, so few accepted his invitation. But Bennett didn't appear to mind. With the straight-backed enthusiasm of a fraternity boy going about a hazing chore, he spent five or ten minutes with just about every woman at the party.

When the phone rang again twenty minutes later, Wendy answered it. It was the infirmary again, and this time Wendy insisted on being given the message if it had anything to do with the unit. "Tell the person in charge that Greta Lampson died, please," the nurse said. "And have the unit supervisor or the social worker call us."

Wendy turned her back to the party. She started to collapse into a chair, but held herself rigid against the desk, not wanting anyone to see her reaction to the news. Greta had not eaten any solid food in more than two months. Doc had predicted that the tube feeding wouldn't keep her alive too long. Wendy choked back her shock and grief and took several slow deep breaths to regain control. She made up her mind to keep the news to herself as long as she could, at least until the patients were in bed for the night. She sucked in a chestful of air, let it out through a muscular smile, and walked out into the party.

A little later, when Henry Dove came up and gave Wendy a hug and said "Thank you, Wendy," she thought she was going to lose it, but she didn't. Another patient, Tom Coolidge, saved her. He was standing next to Henry and he just stuck out his hand, wanting to shake, and said, "I thank ya, too. And I don't have to butter ya up, because I'm gettin' outa this place!"

Wendy shook Tom's hand. He was right. His discharge papers were in the works. He'd probably be getting his bus ticket before winter's end. At least *he* had a chance of making it, Wendy thought.

The phone rang again and Wendy dashed for it, figuring the infirmary was calling back again. Wendy didn't want the bad news to reach anyone else if she could help it.

But it wasn't the infirmary, it was Doc, calling from D-7, where another party was apparently in progress. He said he'd be coming back soon and asked if there were any messages. Wendy said no.

[3]

At 7:10 there was a scream and the crowd went instantly silent. More screams came from the far corner of the dayroom. Rosey and

Ethel Flynn had been sitting on a sofa and Ethel's labor had begun with a splash. Wendy pushed through the crowd and helped Rosey tend to her.

"Let's get her in our wheelchair," Wendy ordered. "If we wait for the infirmary to send one the kid'll be in first grade by the time they get here."

A couple of psych techs from the night shift brought the wheelchair and the sea of people packed into Wilson Cottage parted to let Rosey push Ethel through.

"Breathe!" he urged her, trying to appear calm and doctorly.

"Breathe your ass," Ethel replied, wincing as she rolled out the door.

The party resumed at full speed. Doc returned and could tell right away something was on Wendy's mind. He resolved to ask her about it before he left.

Near eight o'clock, Patty Robito returned and agreed to dance with Bennett Ackerman. A space was cleared in the corner closest to the speakers and they trotted and spun to several Christmas carols.

[4]

After midnight, long after all the guests had left and the remaining patients had gone to bed, Wendy sat alone in the dayroom while the night staff huddled in the nursing station and reminisced about a party whose trash had yet to be taken out. She had told Doc about Greta Lampson, and Doc had nodded. "It was inevitable. Inevitable," he repeated, looking at something far away.

"There's good news, too, sort of," he said. "Alex Greco told me that Zelda Glover assaulted another patient today. She's going to be moved out of here, downstate, to Willowdale."

"I guess that's my Christmas present from the state," Wendy said.

Wendy told Doc about a card she had received from Lily Speere. "She's doing okay, she says. Living at home, you know."

Doc nodded.

"I called to invite her to the party. She didn't come."

Doc shook his head. "I wouldn't have expected her to. She's smart not to. This place isn't exactly like your alma mater, you know. At best it's a kind of purgatory, a limbo, a way station. That's if you're lucky."

After a long silence, Wendy asked Doc if Rosey or anybody had called to tell them how Ethel was doing. Doc shook his head, and said, "Don't worry, Ethel is doing just fine, thank you."

Doc left without asking Wendy what was really on her mind. Wendy didn't volunteer anything, either. Doc's way was to just sit with her and let her talk, and all the time he'd be watching. If she looked like she could handle the next few hours of her life, he was satisfied. Wendy knew that's what he was up to, and could never bring herself to act distraught enough to see what he would do.

It wasn't the next few hours Wendy was worried about, it was the next few dozen years. At around 9:30 Dan Billings had borrowed part of an idea from Bennett Ackerman and had danced Wendy into one of the seclusion rooms and asked her to marry him. She told him she needed some time to think.

Now, in the darkened, party-stained dayroom, Wendy was rehearsing her reply:

"I've decided to go to nursing school."

"I'm not going to have much time to be a wife for a while."

"I'm sorry, Dan."

"Dan, I love you."

The problem Wendy was having was that no matter how she arranged these statements, they didn't add up to a clear No in her heart. And although her desire for this man rattled the foundations of her certainty, she felt that they wouldn't ever add up to anywhere near a No.

[5]

Dr. Steven Rose was having his own problems with yes and no. His head swam in a thick, hot pool of desires and passions, and he suspected the only way to figure this all out was to stop trying to swim.

Ethel Flynn was done with words. She had used words for several months, but didn't need them now. One of the things she had said to him, and had said over and over, was "there's more than thoughts and words." And she was right. Her flesh and the flesh of her newborn son sang a song to Rosey that no words from her lips could compose, and drowned all five of his senses in their liquorous melody.

Rosey touched the glistening skin of Ethel's face and she smiled into his fingers. Her eyes directed his hands and his eyes down to the baby, who sucked hard at her breast.

Rosey wanted to put his mouth on her, too, and when he saw that she knew, he blushed.

Ethel Flynn sighed.

40

[1]

The Thanksgiving open house had gone so well, the staff of D-7 decided to get really ambitious and throw a Christmas party, too. The afternoon of Christmas Eve was chosen, since a few of the higher-functioning patients would be going home for Christmas and there would be relatives coming in all day, anyway. Every member of the staff was responsible for either baking or buying one item of Christmas food to supplement the standard Christmas fare supplied by the hospital kitchen, which would be turkey, again. Many members of the staff weren't sure exactly how the word "again" was being used. Was the sliced turkey served by the hospital merely leftover from Thanksgiving? No one knew for sure except the kitchen staff, and they weren't talking.

Veronia Uyemura brought in several small plum puddings. Timothy Buck was not known for his skill in the kitchen, so he brought three mince pies from the best bakery in Bedloe Valley. Faith Dundee brought in a huge pan of baked yams, with plenty of marshmallows melted on top. Dolores Woods, celebrating Hanuk-kah, baked several batches of cookies in the shape of the Star of David.

In the midst of the preparations, several of the patients were sulking outside the nursing station. Faith was the first to pay atten-tion to this sulking, which was of a different quality than usual. No one was cursing or pulling down his pants or sticking out his tongue while leering at the music therapist.

Faith realized the patients felt left out. She closed the door to the station and proposed to the others that the patients be involved, too. The group decided that was a marvelous idea, and immediately settled the matter of what the patients would supply: a fresh fruit salad.

The wisdom of this idea, relative to the patients' supplying the party with something else, say Christmas cookies, did not descend into common knowledge until, on the day before the party, all the fresh fruit was assembled on two tables in the dayroom and knives had to be handed out to the nine or ten patients who were going to do the work.

"We're handing out knives to them?" Dolores asked, in disbelief.

"How else are we going to go from fresh fruit to fruit salad?" asked Faith.

The patients were eager to get started. One of them was begin-ning to peel a banana, imagining no reason to wait. While the psych techs and Faith and Dolores stared at one another, the patient nonchalantly ate the banana. Following his lead, half of the rest of the group began inspecting the fruit for a suitable snack.

"Call Tim," they decided.

Timothy Buck was called, not so much because they felt his mind would be less fogged, but because in the event of disaster the steps of responsibility would be clearer.

"Just keep an eye on them. Keep track of every knife. Keep them as far apart as the space will allow. We haven't had any stabbings at dinner in three months. I think it'll be okay."

And it was, although for the rest of their lives Faith and Dolores and the psych techs would blanche whenever they saw or smelled or even imagined that fresh fruit was somewhere nearby having its flesh rendered by a paring knife. They would see the sweet life juices flowing and look for it to turn winy red. They would see the glint of stainless steel under fluorescent lights. Most unsettling would be the memory of the intense concentration on the faces of the salad makers, and the eyes that darted under frowns to check if someone was watching. Someone always was, and the fruit salad was accomplished without bloodshed, or even much of a mess. Four patients did later suffer diarrhea from eating too much fruit.

[2]

On Christmas Eve morning, patients and day staff of D-7 found the unit transformed. The night staff had brought in decorations to supplement the stale ornaments supplied by the hospital. There were Christmas bells and a small silver-foil tree festooned with blue glass balls. Day staff brought their own decorations to add to what the night elves had left. At first they decided against cardboard angels, not wishing to reinforce any of the patients' delusions. Dr. Uyemura overruled the ban, however. "This week, we all believe in angels, okay?" she said.

The patients were dressed in fresh, clean clothes—new ones, when available. The worst moments were in the morning when the bathroom was crowded with patients taking extra long to shave and wash and generally primp for the big day. The psych techs aborted a nascent fistfight by running between two men and shouting "It's Christmas! It's Christmas!"

Tables were set up and the food brought in sooner than planned because the staff had word that some relatives were coming early to pick up their patients and leave. Many did come early, but no one seemed to leave early. Night staff came in the middle of the day and admitted it was because they didn't want to miss this for anything. Fran and Brad Channing arrived around three, and all the relatives who were expected to come were there by four.

Dolores thought it was no accident that the most normally unmanageable patients seemed to have the most avid dedication to singing, so she had corralled every one of them for the unit choir and trained them for weeks on a single carol, "Silent Night." Staff, or anyone who happened down the hall or past one of the open or few broken windows of D-7, were greeted by a multiharmonied, uneven-rhythmed version of the carol. These qualities did not change over the weeks. If anything, the choir became somewhat more sure of their many harmonies and varied rhythms, so the resulting song owned a vitality that lifted and swept every listener into a Christmas mood. And if the voices didn't do it, the earnest concentration illuminating the faces of the singers did.

Alex Greco made an appearance at the party with Doc, and both men joined with the choir for three choruses. Alex had planned to take Fran Channing and other members of the Family Organization aside and tell them he had not been named superintendent. But he decided to sing another chorus of "Silent Night" instead and call them on the phone during the following week.

Through the afternoon, several psychiatrists and assorted staff from around the hospital peeked in. All the food disappeared by six o'clock. The fruit salad went first, perhaps because every patient who had wielded a knife made sure every person knew he had made the salad, "so you better taste it before it's gone."

One patient was lost, but soon found lying on his bed in a profound depression. No relative had come to see him. He had not seen a member of his family in almost a decade. But another patient gave him his sack of hospital-supplied "gifts" and the depression lifted enough for him to come back out to the party and complain about how the fruit salad was gone before he even had a chance to taste it.

No one wanted to be the first to leave, but the family who had the farthest to drive finally took a psych tech aside and asked for their son's backpack. They were escorted out by the psych tech, who came back and said the air had that pregnant dampness of a coming snow. More familes left. By 7:30 only staff and hospital-bound patients remained. The party chugged forward on momentum. Staff from other units joined what was left of the choir and sang more choruses of "Silent Night." The hospital kitchen sent over more food.

The remnants and mess had a cheery life all their own. Long into the night, even after all the patients were asleep, staff held off from cleaning up until the last snowy breaths of night whispered in the dawn.

41

George Konopski had been spending Christmas Eve with a ward full of violent, mentally ill men for several years now, and if truth were told, he had volunteered to do it. There was no way they were going to leave the V-units without regular staff, so that meant at least two of the regular crew had to be there. Konopski, as commander in chief, couldn't expect the men to take this duty without his showing up, too. This is what Konopski told his wife, anyway, when she complained about his missing another Christmas Eve with the family.

Of course, his wife wasn't buying any of it, not even if he threw in something about Alex Greco asking him to do it. Konopski's wife knew that Alex Greco was as crazy as her husband was, and that he would be at the hospital on Christmas Eve, too. One year she had refused to accept George's stock excuses, not because she didn't know the real answer, but because she wanted him to admit it.

"Okay, you got me," he said. "I just can't stand the thought of those poor bastards locked up in that place on Christmas Eve."

Of course, not all of them were alone. More than a few had girlfriends or wives who showed up with sad little cakes or warped cookies. They wanted to have a party, but Konopski always had to put the kibosh on that action. There was no way they could turn the V-units into a dance hall, even if every patient had a female partner. "The guy running the unit before me tried it," Konopski said. "Turned the freaking place into a dance hall. Had patients dancing with other men, some with their girlfriends. Well, before you know it, some guy wanted to cut in. And who's pinching whose ass or calling who a fairy! Christ, they had to call in every cop in the hospital, and they were cleaning up blood and glass for a week! Some Christmas Eve!"

Some of the couples tried to sneak off to the dormitory or seclusion rooms. This was a tough call, especially since some of the men were not your average boys next door when it came to sexual hang-ups and fantasies. Normally, some of the men got involved with each other, and, if they didn't get violent or hurt each other, the staff usually looked the other way. So, on Christmas Eve, the dormitory was placed off limits because it was so difficult to monitor, but two seclusion rooms were reserved for trysts. There was seldom any trouble with this arrangement. The women were pretty good at handling their men, and the staff kept the curious away from the seclusion rooms.

This year was no exception, in fact it was quieter than most. Only five women showed up, and one of them came for a patient who had been discharged back to the state prison weeks ago. She was friendly and easygoing, however, and quickly took up with a patient who had been best friends with her boyfriend.

Normally, Konopski would have been home by midnight, but this was not a normal year. This year Konopski wasn't going to get home until Christmas morning, for not only had he agreed to take the long shift in the V-units, but he had also said yes when a friend asked him to fill in for her in the geriatric unit.

Of all the wards at the hospital, of all the possible wards in all the possible mental hospitals, the geriatric unit was the only one that gave Konopski the creeps. "That place is too quiet and too clean. It's spooky," he said. It wasn't that you could actually point to any specific area of the unit that was cleaner than the best-kept unit elsewhere. The floors and walls in G-5 just seemed to sparkle with a

surreal luster. Maybe it had something to do with the silence.
Except for an occasional moan or grunt, or when the background
hum of a respirator became audible, the G-unit was quiet as a tomb.
Perhaps the brain registered noise in the same cells as clutter and
dirt, and when those cells were overstimulated, as they were in
every other ward at Bedloe, and then absolutely ignored, as they
were in the G unit, well, the result was a distortion of natural
consciousness.

All of the patients in G-5 were at least sixty-five years old and
severely ill in some way that had obliterated most of the normal
expressions of intelligence. They were not simply old schizophrenics or manic-depressives or schizoaffectives. They might have
been at one time, but all now had advanced organic disease, which
meant that their nervous systems were in shambles. Many had been
patients at Bedloe since they were children. Some had lived more
or less normal lives until their illnesses became advanced and
intolerable to those around them. All but a few now spent their
entire lives in bed, some in huge, adult-size steel hospital cribs. The
more active among them, maybe half a dozen at any given time,
were able to sit in a chair during the day. Three were able to hobble
around the unit with the aid of aluminum walkers.

Turnover in G-5 was not what one would expect. In fact, the unit's
patient turnover was no higher than any other at the hospital, and its
staff turnover was far and away the lowest. There was something
ghoulish about that fact. Konopski wondered about how anyone
could stand to work in this place every day, where all discharges
were to the hospital morgue. Konopski figured it must be because it
was the easiest unit to work in. No violence. No arguments.

When Konopski looked into the patients' eyes, what disturbed
him most was their intense concentration on something he could
not see or imagine, as if each woman or man was working at some
secret, personal task. Konopski would have rejoiced at some eye
contact, some recognition, even a malevolent leer as he often
received in the V-unit. But whatever these patients were about, they
could not share it or reveal it. And behind those busy stares,
nothing, a wall—as if their faces were posters.

It was so quiet and so calm that there was nothing to distract you
from whatever junk was weighing on your mind. In the V-unit, you
had to concentrate on what was going around you or you might get

clobbered. In here, there was nothing going on around you, so your thoughts ruled the silence.

What made it even worse was the psych techs kept to themselves, so anything but the most necessary conversation was out. Konopski figured they picked up on how spooked he was.

So instead of running down a list of Christmas presents, Konopski unwrapped his catalog of worries and woes. The one nice thing about sitting out the night in G-5 was that he didn't have Linus Dillinger staring at him with his confident smile that was half frown.

It didn't look like the new administration was going to forget about Dillinger. They weren't as nasty about it as Akbar had been, but they made it clear that it was part of Konopski's job description. Sure, it would be easy enough for Konopski to examine him and pronounce him sane, or insane. Either way he'd be agreeing with at least half a dozen other psychiatrists. But that wouldn't be the end of it. It was going to be a lawyer party no matter what he said.

Maybe the problem wasn't Dillinger or the lawyers, but the job, after all. Everything was uniformly dark, and seeming darker despite the holiday and the sparkle of G-5. The FBI had finally come through on Tang. Not that it would have saved his life, but he had been a soldier, some kind of special forces unit, and his whole family had been wiped out before his eyes. He had been in and out of military hospitals, sometimes discharged, sometimes AWOL. Konopski had stopped reading the report before he found out whether the man had been AWOL when he was brought to Bedloe. Somebody else would take care of that, somebody who enjoyed playing with records.

Tang's ghost was joined by Ned Salmon's. Ned had been picked up again, this time for throwing a bale of newspapers at a police car. The record said "assaulting officers." Ned never even got before a judge. His "assault" took place on a Sunday morning and he was thrown into a holding cell, bawling like a baby, the record noted. He was found dead the next morning, broken neck. Cops still hadn't figured out how little Ned had managed to break his own neck without a rope or a belt. The other men in the holding cell were equally mystified.

Well, Konopski thought, add one more unsolved mystery to a long, long list.

There was a small television in the nursing station, and Konopski was about to turn it on when he heard people coming in from outside. Two women wrapped in black wool coats entered through the swinging doors with a swirl of cold. They were middle-aged, maybe late forties. Sisters, Konopski could tell. The gray in their eyebrows and around their temples gave a kind of misty appearance to their faces.

They approached the station talking softly to each other, and didn't turn to address Konopski until they were right in front of him. "We're here to visit Mr. Romanov," the taller one said.

Konopski reached for the directory and started searching for the whereabouts of that patient.

"We're his daughters," the other one said.

Konopski found the room number and came out from behind the counter to escort them to the room, more from curiosity than procedure. He remembered something one of the psych techs said about some visitors coming later on. He looked at his watch: it was almost midnight.

As they walked down the hall, the sisters' heels echoed. They kept their eyes straight ahead and did not peek into any of the other rooms as they passed. One of them carried a red foil-wrapped box.

"Here's your father's room," Konopski said.

"Same room as last year," the tall one said as they walked in and gave the room a quick inspection. The room seemed swathed in blue light, and on the bed was a bundle of blue sheets and shadows. The tall one walked up to the bed and gently pulled back the sheet. Konopski felt a chill at the sight of the shrunken man in fetal position on the bed. Against the tufts of white hair, his skin appeared flushed a bright orange-pink. Mr. Romanov stared straight ahead with diligent crystal-blue eyes.

Konopski didn't want to leave, so he picked up the old man's chart and inspected it. "Everything looks okay." he said, authoritatively. "Pretty stable." The woman seemed to ignore him as they pulled chairs over and took up stations in front of their father.

"Dad's been stable for almost twenty years," the tall one said as she took off her coat. "He's been at this hospital for seventeen years, and in this ward for fifteen."

"I see," Konopski said.

"Hi, Dad. Merry Christmas," the shorter woman said as she

leaned over, brushed her father's hair back and kissed him on his bare forehead. The old man blinked, but that was all.

The tall sister moved in and did the same. "We brought you your favorite chocolates, Dad. Here you go." She placed the red-foil box in front of her father on the bed. No response.

"One year, I guess it was about four or five Christmases ago, he reached out and grabbed it. First time that happened. He used to love these before he got sick. He'd go out and buy them by the case, give everyone in the family a box, in addition to their presents." She turned from Konopski to her father, who was still staring straight ahead and whose hands were still tucked between his knees. She reached over and picked up the box and unwrapped it.

"See, Dad, your favorite!" she chirped mechanically. It was a box of chocolate-covered cherries, and she now had the box open and was offering one to the man on the bed.

"C'mon, Suse, you know he can't," the other sister said. "Don't tease him."

"Okay, okay. Here, Dad." She placed the candy against his lips. The old man shuddered and jerked. His lip quivered and started to grasp the chocolate and pull it into his mouth. His eyes opened wider, as brown and then red juice dripped down the side of his face. He moaned and slobbered and stuck his tongue out, dropping the gooey mess on the bed. The daughter picked it up in a tissue and flung it into a wastebasket by the bed. Then she took out a fresh candy and started over.

"Here you go, Pop." Konopski knew it was time to leave, but he was transfixed. The mess on the bed got worse and worse, and the thought crossed his mind that there might be some problem with this on the patient's chart. He wasn't on intravenous feeding, so Konopski put the chart back and decided it didn't make any difference.

"We don't even know, for sure, if he knows we're here," the tall sister said.

"Probably not," the other said, defensively, as she fed her father another chocolate-covered cherry.

"Oh, you never know," the other replied. "We come every Christmas, that's all. Once a year."

"We don't know why we do. We just do. To remind us."

"Every year we figure it will be the last. But he just lives another year," she said, with an air of practiced strength.

"He was always a strong man," the other said.

Both sisters took deep breaths and held on to them. Konopski realized they might be holding themselves for his benefit, so he nodded and left. "I'll be back at the station if you need anything."

"Thank you, Doctor," they said in unison.

As Konopski walked up the hall toward the station, he heard the two women start to sing a Christmas carol in harmony that was hushed, but clear as a church bell on a cold night.

They kept on singing, and when the psych techs came back from their break and turned on the television, Konopski fled its inane squawking and carried a chair down the hall and sat outside the room where the sisters were singing to their father.

42

Alex drove home from the hospital that evening wondering how many more times in his life he would be doing it. He wanted to forget the hospital, to leave it behind the stone wall, with miles and miles of cold air between him and its daily round of exertions and frustrations.

He couldn't shake either his anger or his distress over the appointment of another bureaucrat to the superintendent's position. Maybe it's karma, Alex mused, half seriously. Physicians brought this upon themselves and upon the society by their "high and mighty" attitude, by acting as if they were gods, demanding powers and privileges and accepting little accountability.

Yes, that was true. That was certainly true, Alex agreed. But who else accepted this role, this warrior priesthood? Not the priests and ministers. They had given up the real battle against chaos and turned their attention elsewhere. How many families in agony had Alex talked to who had first gone to their clergyman for help when madness began making forays into their family life? He figured about half, although the statistics said something like 40 percent went to their clergy first—and most hit a dead end.

So who was there to accept the role? Who but physicians came forward to really minister to matters of life and death, pain and misery, and the struggle of the mind to escape the typhoon from which it was born? Whatever miracle had created organized consciousness apparently could not be taken for granted. It was a miracle that had to be recreated over and over again. And sometimes the machinery of creation failed. The Enemy got inside the gates, took prisoners of loving memories, made casualties of dreams.

Did the clergymen tell the families it was "God's will"?

Alex sometimes wondered if he wasn't, indeed, battling against God's will, for he felt he was struggling against the very lines of definition of the universe, the violent edge where things are made and unmade, where the distinct and logical merges with the chaotic. He was grabbing souls that had slipped off the edge, trying to drag them back, and losing most of them. Even if he should be able to save all he touched, there were multitudes sliding across the boundaries he never even saw, let alone touched. But he knew they were there, because the battle line went on forever.

At the D-7 party, Fran Channing had come up to him and asked him if he had any news about his mentally ill daughter. Alex confessed he had not had a call from Carmen in several weeks.

Fran saw the pain in his face when Alex spoke of his daughter, and said to him, "I've wanted to say this to you for some time, but . . . I just couldn't, Dr. Greco. Now I am going to say it. When you told us about your daughter, you said you couldn't do anything for her. You were wrong about that. You do a lot for her. You love her. You love her so much it hurts you. And you will never stop loving her, no matter how much it hurts."

She started to say something else, but was called away by her husband, who wanted to gather up their son and leave. But the damage had been done. Alex's anger and fear were shattered, swept away by his shame, leaving a clear surface of grief.

There was only that, he realized, only that touching with the hand, that looking with the eyes, that saving wish. He could add the prayer of a drug, the sword of a lightning bolt, and whatever other weapons were placed before him. But no one suffered or fought more for their loved ones than Fran Channing and the others. Alex was one of them, and would always be.

Now Alex kept the Lincoln just over the speed limit, with an image in his head of what his home looked like. The lights would be on in every room and Maria would have the children dressed up and fidgeting around the place, making and removing messes of wrapping paper, food, and toys. Alex wondered if she would remember to tie the big red bow on the front gate.

That's the way it was. The house was a glowing star on the street. The red bow was where it should be, and Alex was immediately swamped by a squall of children the moment he was in the front door. Maria called from the kitchen. Alex found her leaning over a cookbook.

If the Greco household had any traditions, one was that every Christmas Maria would set a table burdened under a mass of Christmas goodies. Later, staring at the remains of that table, Alex felt a little dizzy and a little glad at the richness of his life. He hummed a Christmas carol.

Another Greco tradition was to be indecisive about whether to open presents before going to bed or in the morning. Maria usually was the strict constructionist on this issue, and favored waiting until morning. Alex usually cast his vote for getting it over with so everyone could sleep late. The children, of course, were prepared not to sleep. But this year Alex sided with Maria, although he didn't tell her why. He wanted the feeling of greedy anticipation in the house to last all night. He wanted to lie awake and bathe in it, and rise at first light with the same ravenous expectations as the children. Nothing would get in the way of this, not the moonless night, not sleep, not even the telephone call that came near midnight. Alex answered before it woke up Maria.

"Hey, Dad."

"Hiya, Carmen."

"Sorry I called so late."

"It's okay. Where are ya?"

"At Grandma's. Lotsa food. You know."

"That's good. That's good."

"I ate a lot, Dad."

"It's good for you."

"Hey, Dad?"

"Yeah, Carmen?"

"Dad . . . Merry Christmas."

Alex drew a silent deep breath and held on to it.

"Dad?"

"Merry Christmas, Baby."

The clicks at the end of the connection echoed in Alex's head for a while after he put the phone down, and he wondered if he would sleep, and if he would sleep, if the dream would come, and if it did, if he would see Carmen in it.

43

Fran took a hot shower to relax before going to bed. By the time she got to bed Brad was in glorious dreamland, which was just as well. She didn't want her tossing and turning to keep the poor man awake, with all the driving he'd done today, to the hospital and then back with Walter.

With Walter. Walter was in the house now. Fran reached out with her senses to find him in the silence, to feel his presence. It was a nice Christmas present. Fran held back from making it more than that, although she knew she had plenty of feelings about it straining to break loose and explode its significance. Walter had made progress, had gotten a little better. He could keep getting better, or he could get worse. Or both, up and down, back and forth, a step forward and a step back.

Fran figured this crazy dance engendered a dizzy sense of terror because it tilted her off her expectations. So the secret was to have only one expectation, one hope. She made that her prayer: *I will do all I can.*

Fran said a prayer for herself, for Walter, for Brad, for Alex Greco, and for other Family Organization members.

Outside, the air was growing heavy and still with the cold, and Fran could feel the chill around the window, through both layers of glass. She tugged on the blankets to free them from the tangle around Brad's feet.

She heard something and froze, holding the blankets a foot above her. When she was sure of the silence, she let them down.

Then she heard it again, the sound of the floor creaking. Someone was walking or standing in another part of the house.

There was a clunk from Walter's room. Fran shivered.

With the next clunk there came a ringing and a buzzing of guitar strings, and Fran felt the life in her body poise itself for flight. She wrapped her pillow around her ears and forced her breathing loudly through her nose to block the sounds. She squeezed her eyes shut.

I'll do all I can. I'll do all I can, Fran repeated inwardly. *I'll do all I can, please let him go to sleep.*

The repetitive twanging stopped. When Fran felt relieved enough to stop pressing the pillow to her ears, she acknowledged that it hadn't been as bad as she thought it would be. He would go to sleep, now.

There was another clunk from Walter's room, and Fran tensed again, ready to bury herself in the bed. She kept her eyes shut.

A clear chord sounded. Then another. Then the first few tentative notes of a melody.

Silence.

The chord again. Clear and bright.

This could be a dream, or I could be dead, Fran thought. But when she heard the guitar again, and recognized the simple tune, she opened her eyes wide and looked around the room and saw that she was alive in the darkness and the music was real.

EPILOGUE

In May, Wendy Dixon married Dan Billings under a magnolia tree in full glory at Poe Lake. The patients and staff of Wilson Cottage attended. Doc gave the bride away. Lily Speere was maid of honor. In the fall, Wendy began nursing school while maintaining a full-time schedule at Bedloe.

Doc reached an out-of-court settlement with the hospital and came back to work in June. The identities of the men who assaulted him were never discovered.

Lily Speere got a part-time job as a waitress and began writing poetry. A small Midwestern literary journal accepted three of her poems for publication. She was offered a scholarship to a southern university, which she accepted.

Dr. Steven Rose and Ethel Flynn were married in a civil ceremony three days after her discharge from Bedloe State Hospital in September. Rosey began a special residency in family practice while Ethel got a job as a topless dancer.

Bennett Ackerman managed to hang on to his "heavy hat" until October, when he gave it up voluntarily.

Zelda Glover, the patient who attacked Wendy, remained seriously ill in a locked ward for violent women patients at Willowdale State Hospital.

George Konopski resigned from Bedloe State Hospital in February and got a job as a "contract" psychiatrist at a community mental health center. A week after he left the hospital, the patient who had earlier begged, and then demanded, drugs from him repeated the performance with Konopski's replacement. The psychiatrist relented and was immediately brought up on charges before the medical quality review board. The charges were dismissed when it was discovered that the paperwork for the hearing and the report by the undercover officer for the state department of mental health—the patient who had asked for the drugs—referred to the psychiatrist as "George Konopski."

Linus Dillinger was examined by a psychiatrist hired by the attorney general's office, pronounced sane, and sent back to death row. A massive legal battle began. All parties to the case, except George Konopski and Alex Greco, were either sued or called as witnesses. Legal experts commenting on the case expected it to last for at least a decade.

The murderer of the woman patient from D-7 was never found.

Dr. Dean Lester, fired from D-7 by Alex Greco, was hired by the Veterans Administration.

In the spring, Timothy Buck began to receive telephone threats related to his reform work on unit D-7. In June he quit Bedloe State Hospital. Work on the Bedloe farm ceased.

Dr. Veronica Uyemura, Dan Billings, Faith Dundee, Dolores Woods, and the rest of the staff continued to improve conditions on the unit, despite similar threats. As much as they did, they knew they weren't doing enough.

Fran Channing continued her support of her son and became an officer in the Family Organization. Walter Channing brought his guitar back to the hospital after his Christmas furlough and, with the help of Faith and Dolores, started a band composed entirely of patients.

Losing his bid for superintendent was at once a bitter disappointment and a sweet breeze of liberation for Alex Greco. He resigned from Bedloe State Hospital. He and his family moved to Montana, where he became the director and only psychiatrist in a small county clinic, and where he managed to sandwich in administrative duties while seeing six to ten patients a day. Alex made progress on the painting of his dream. The calls from Carmen continued.

Sam Akbar disappeared into the state bureaucracy. Although the new superintendent and medical director of Bedloe State Hospital allowed the continuation of many of the reforms begun by Alex Greco, the staff of D-7, and the Family Organization, he did not stimulate many new changes. Morale at the hospital began to slide when 10 percent of the staff was laid off.

Toward the end of the year, the governor and legislature slashed tens of millions of dollars from the budget for the care of the mentally ill. One third of the clinics serving the mentally ill across the state were closed, and there were rumblings in the state Department of Mental Health about closing Bedloe State Hospital.